CW01084292

The Sealed Box of Suicide

Colin Tatz · Simon Tatz

The Sealed Box of Suicide

The Contexts of Self-Death

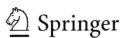 Springer

Colin Tatz
Australian National University
Canberra, ACT, Australia

Simon Tatz
Curtin, ACT, Australia

ISBN 978-3-030-28158-8   ISBN 978-3-030-28159-5   (eBook)
https://doi.org/10.1007/978-3-030-28159-5

This Springer imprint is published by the registered company Springer Nature Switzerland AG
The registered company address is: Gewerbestrasse 11, 6330 Cham, Switzerland

In memory
of
great-uncle (and great-great uncle) Dotke,
who talked and looked like a poet
but sold chicken-feed instead;
a bad book-keeper,
he took his life
because he misread his healthy credit column
—as a debit.

Acknowledgements

Writing a book about suicide, and having something new to say, is a tough business. The men and women we thank have helped with grace and kindness. A few have commented on ideas, assumptions and judgments. Several provided sources.

Our warmest thanks to Hannah Andrevski, Vicken Babkenian, Michael Barnes, Douglas Booth, Amanda Bresnan, Belinda Carpenter, Alain Coltier, Panayiotis Diamadis, Michael Diamond, Armen Gakavian, Meher Grigorian, Gillian Heller, Herbert Herzog, Ian Hickie, Winton Higgins, Wendy Johnson, Michael Kral, Margaret Macallister, Ian Marsh, John Mendoza, Jessica Palmer, Nicole Roberts, Michael Robertson, David Robinson, Alan Rosen, Kim Ryan, Jennifer Schultz Moore, Said Shahtahmasebi, Linda Shields, Gordon Tait, Akiva Tatz, Corey Tatz, Karen Tatz, Paul Tatz, Tracey Westerman, Asher Westropp-Evans, Jennifer White and Lesley Yee.

Sebastian Rosenberg reviewed the entire manuscript, made critical and useful comments, added sources and helped shape the final text. We heeded his wisdom. Ross Mellick gave us several throwaway lines that became long paragraphs. Michael Dudley provided significant sources and suggestions. Pam Tatz sorted out the citations and footnotes. Sandra Tatz gave her sage advice, time and editing skills to this project. Shinjini Chatterjee, Jayanthi Krishnamoorthi and Muruga Prashanth Rajendran handled the book's production with great style.

A special thanks to Belinda Carpenter and Gordon Tait who brought Colin Tatz into the team that was awarded an Australian Research Grant award, DP 150101402, 'Investigating the coronial determination of suicide as a category of death', 2015–2019.

Contents

About the Authors

Colin Tatz was Professor of Politics at the University of New England and Macquarie University in Australia. He is now an honorary lecturer in Politics and International Relations at the Australian National University. His books treat comparative race politics, Aboriginal affairs, genocide studies, migration, suicide and sports history.

Simon Tatz has been Director of Communications (Mental Health Australia), Director of Public Health (Australian Medical Association), Manager of Media and Marketing (ACT Health), Director of Policy (Mental Health Victoria), Chief of Staff (Minister for Higher Education) and a policy and media adviser in the Australian Parliament.

Chapter 1
Explanations

Suicides often, by the very nature of their death in our society,
put their skeletons in their survivors' closets.

—Edwin Shneidman [American clinical psychologist and
suicidologist, 1918–2009]

Suicide is a form of murder – premeditated murder. It isn't
something you do the first time you think of doing it. It takes
getting used to. And you need the means, the opportunity, the
motive. A successful suicide demands good organisation and a
cool head, both of which are usually incompatible with the
suicidal state of mind.

—Susanne Kaysen [American novelist]

Abstract The purpose of the book is to examine why society reacts so strongly and so badly to suicide; to evoke fresh thinking about a taboo by bringing to light the external and contextual factors that impinge on self-death; to canvass the conventional biomedical model of suicide as illness.

Keywords Provocation · Spurs to this book · Social change

Readers need to know what this book is and what it isn't.

It is not a textbook but it could be instructive for the professionals who deal with suicide and for the families who have lost a member. We hope that it speaks to a public that is curious or simply interested in finding out more about this bewildering behaviour. The book is not a polemic in the diatribe sense, nor an attack on the medical profession and the suicide prevention agencies. Some may read it that way and some will do so, but to question, even sharply, is not to attack. It is not a treatise on suicide theory, nor a research essay based on systematic investigation (apart from the chapter on Australian coroners and aspects of Australian Aboriginal genocide). It is not the outcome of a set of clipboard questionnaire responses. It is not based

© Springer Nature Switzerland AG 2019
C. Tatz and S. Tatz, *The Sealed Box of Suicide*,
https://doi.org/10.1007/978-3-030-28159-5_1

on official suicide statistics and their analyses, much of which is dubious rather than contentious. In no way is it a belittling of religious beliefs.

The essence of suicide, if it is to be found, requires looking at individual cases and circumstances, not in official figures. But this is a critical work that examines the merits and faults of professions that purport to comprehend the nature of suicide and insist they can prevent the phenomenon.

While suicide has been part of the human experience in most cultures, the biomedical world has managed to imprison suicide for more than a century. Supporters of that vision of health have come to portray the behaviour as an 'epidemic', a scourge, a blight and a 'curse' on our society, an inevitable outcome of mental illness, certainly of depression. No longer the domain of philosophers, poets, priests and lawyers, medicine has command of a behaviour that used to be customary, traditional and very normal. Suicide is so much more than a manner of death. It has, as American scholar Jack Douglas tells us, social meanings (Douglas 1967). As such, there is space enough to cope with some new suggestions, ideas and judgements about a topic so overwhelmingly simplified, unhelpfully boxed in as 'depression = suicidal thoughts = medication'.

Is the study of suicide a science? Through the travails and sorrows of his tragic character Werther, the great German writer Johann Wolfgang van Goethe (1749–1832) insisted that suicide is part of human nature. Each generation, he reminded us, needs to come to terms with this reality. Based on that perspective, the controversial Hungarian-American psychiatrist Thomas Szasz (1920–2012) was adamant that suicide is a moral issue: 'Dying voluntarily is a choice intrinsic to human existence. It is our ultimate, 'fatal freedom'' (Szasz 1998). The French sociologist Jean Baechler defined suicide as 'a human privilege' (Baechler 1979: 42). The French novelist and philosopher Albert Camus (1913–1960) declared that 'there is only one really serious philosophical problem and that is suicide' (Camus 1955).

Suicide is unquestionably a moral, philosophical and existential matter. But, despite extensive efforts, the study of suicide is *not* a province of science. Assuredly, it is not capable of systematic observation and experiment lending itself to empirical measurement, analysis, replication and validation. The most studied of all human behaviours, libraries of journals and monographs examine suicide and go to great methodological lengths in search of measurable criteria to explain it. Certainly, patterns can be discerned, impressions gained, theories developed and disciplinary perspectives pondered. But regression coefficients, chi-square correlations and age-standardised rates notwithstanding, what, for example, do we learn from a table that tells us that the suicide rate for two decades (1970–1990) across several nations varied as follows: Hungary at 39.9 deaths per 100,000 of the population, Denmark 24.1, Australia 23.6, Spain 7.7, Italy 7.5, Chile 5.6, Greece 3.5 and Mexico 2.3 (Lester 1996: 100)? Is it really likely that Magyars in Hungary are 17 times more prone to suicide than Mexicans? These statistics don't tell us how much these comparisons depend on the differences in registering and reporting between national practices, given the widespread belief in Catholic and Eastern Orthodox nations that suicide is both a sin and a taboo subject. And the Danish figure completely masks the fact that Greenland Inuit, whether on home soil or in Denmark, have a rate of 83 per 100,000—among the world's highest figure (WHO 2011).

Reporting/registering criteria differ markedly, even in a small population country like Australia, with its federal system of governance and its eight separate coronial jurisdictions.[1] The British–American social scientist Lester (1996: 11) reported on a study of 40 case files presented to coroners in eight countries, with no significant difference between their verdicts. 'Coroner biases are not related to national suicide rates', he concluded. That was hardly a controlled laboratory test, and one has to ask serious questions about national cultures, ruling religious canons and suicide reporting before one can accept those rates as statistical 'gospel'. In the Australian research study discussed in Chap. 11, we show how inconsistent the determination of suicide is across the Australian jurisdictions. Herein lies an inherent flaw in suicide studies, namely, the acceptance of official reports—the very bases on which practically all suicidology rests—as realistic, reliable and comparable. Our contention is that no reputable science can operate on premises or baselines such as these. Further, statistics have yet to show that their analysis produces a better *understanding* of suicide than examination of individual case studies.

Suicide is fraught with faith, fear, folklore, demonology, dogma, dread, mystery, secrecy and speculation. Given the myriad conjectures and suppositions surrounding the behaviour, we offer several insights based on three decades of limping towards a contextual anthropology of suicide among Australian Aboriginal youth, a group within which suicide was unknown half a century ago and in which it is now rampant (Tatz 2005). That kind of anthropology is not hard science but rests rather on, among other things, observation, participant observation, and the intuitive knowledge and understanding of the meaning of an action from the actor's point of view. Based on the concept of German sociologist and philosopher Max Weber (1864–1920), it is called *verstehen* in German (Dilthey 1989).

Most critical analyses provoke responses from those who see value only in the past and immediate present. In which case, this book is a positive provocation—not to incur anger but to stimulate thinking outside the sealed box in which suicide is confined. In an ironic sense, this book is something of an inquest, an inquisitorial look at why suicide creates such angst and anger, even hysteria, when compared to homicide and other violent causes of death. The text examines, at some length, why a century or more of prevention activity has not worked and why there can be no vaccination against self-elected death. Intervention in crisis time is something quite different. The medical profession, and those who specialise in psychiatry (and psychology), has been addressing suicide for over two centuries now, and have yet to unlock the enigma of why the living choose to die.

---

[1] Each of six states and two territories has its own coronial system, as discussed in Chap. 11 of this book. But there is a cross-jurisdictional committee attempting to create national consistency in reporting, definitions, involving health personnel, coroners and police.

We offer suggestions about alleviating suicide, activities that deflect the immediacy of ending one's life. We look at the professions of coroner and doctor and ponder their levels of tuition about suicide. In the book, and in the final chapter particularly, we discuss some 32 topics that bear directly on suicide but which are almost always left out of the conversations. Hopefully, the book will be a gainful road to comprehension (and perhaps an accommodation) of why people kill themselves.

Our intellectual traditions, and certainly the professions—like medicine, law, architecture, accountancy and engineering—don't like untidiness. Neat laws, formulae, rules and principles govern their working lives by providing order and reasonably predictable outcomes. Suicide is the enemy of tidiness, of conformity, of scientific truths. Rarely are there predicting signs of an intent to take a life, of attempts to end life, of doing so. (Later we discuss research that has found family awareness of signs that are not reported to health care professionals). Shock and bewilderment are common responses to suicide, indicative of the unexpectedness of the deed, the violence inherent in the act of cessation, the dying so suddenly and so quickly.

A new tidiness has entered coronial practice in England. Until now coroners there have had to prove suicide beyond a reasonable doubt (98–99%). The British High Court has ruled (in the *James Maughan* case, 2018) that a balance of probabilities, 51%, will suffice. Given the serious under-reporting of suicide over the decades, the new standard of proof will likely double the existing rates, perhaps even treble them. Other jurisdictions, such as Australia, have used the 51% standard for some time now, and that lower standard has a significant impact on official rates. In sum, there is a great deal more suicide than we believed to be the case.

On hearing that we were working on this book, an immediate response was 'but you're not doctors! You're not psychiatrists!' Such indignation tells us where Western society is on the matter of suicide—it is deemed to be, implacably believed to be, *solely* in the medical domain. But suicide is not the sole province of medicine. In Australia, at least, there are three or four tiers of persons who deal with the matter: they range from the 12-year trained psychiatrist to the thousands of formally untrained persons involved in non-government organisation (NGO) activity as 'preventionists' of suicide. Why that is so and why it shouldn't be so is a major theme of this volume by two seemingly unlikely authors. One is an elderly academic versed in political science, public administration, sociology and law. The other is a social science graduate, a mid-life administrator with long service as a federal political parliamentary staffer and in medical and mental health agencies. They are father and son. Suicide is hardly the exclusive right of any one -ology, any one set of lenses among the many that come under the umbrella of science. There is a science of birth and death; there is also an art of living and dying.

The impetus for the fascination with suicide comes from several sources. One was the discovery that at least ten members of our relatively small family had taken their lives, a remarkable statistic. Another was that a great-uncle, a grain merchant, had confused his accounting ledgers (thin cardboard sheets folded into eight leaves), and wrongly believing he was bankrupt, adjourned to his adjacent barn and hanged himself with his trouser braces. Uncle 'D' wasn't mentally ill: he simply couldn't face the ignominy of insolvency, a monumental *shanda*, shame, in his day, age and context. The point of his story is not just his death, but that it took the family almost 50 years to reveal his manner of death, the skeleton in our closet. Yet another prompt was the research finding that there was no suicide in Australian Aboriginal life before 1960—after which came an irruption that placed several communities among the highest rates on the planet. Why? had to be the obvious response.

Cesare Pavese, a noted Italian poet and social critic, once wrote that no one ever lacked a reason for suicide. We believe that. We also accept fully the neuroscientific verdict that reason and emotion are both indicators of *thinking* that both travel the same neural pathways in the brain. Does a suicider—the term we use for the actor—*think*? Do they form an intent, however wrong an intent society deems it to be? In an hallucinatory state, a person may believe they can fly and jump from an apartment balcony. But, for the most part, the suicider has a reason and it is the inability to fathom it that both confronts and affronts society. Suicide runs counter to the truism that 'life is precious'.

The suicider is the agent of their demise, and it is a reasonable assumption that the medical profession should focus on the 'inside' of that agency in order to find out why that pathway was chosen (Broz and Münster 2016; Douglas 1967). But the agent can never be devoid of context, that is, an 'outside' existence that involves a social setting, a physical place, a set of relationships, a cultural and religious milieu, a welter of connections that give one a sense of belonging. For many, for the million who commit suicide every year, their outside world goes awry; their centres fall apart and cannot hold together. At present, there is an obstacle: those who look inside have little if any training in looking outside, and to date, the inside vision has shown itself incapable of putting a stop to self-cessation. Even those few with inside/outside skills find it extremely difficult to 'engineer' solutions for those displaying suicidal symptoms.

There is always some room for optimism. Social change can be inordinately slow, and sometimes it can happen in a rush. Smoking was an indelible norm, was then implicated in cancer and finally is accepted as the killer that it clearly is. Divorce was once rare and deplored, but today the rate is between 38 and 50% in Canada, the UK and the USA—a strange but common badge of dubious 'pride'. Homosexuality was always an abomination in the eyes of many religions and became a mental disorder in the eyes of American psychiatry in the middle of the last century. Today we celebrate same-sex marriages. Suicide was, in turn, a form of badness, madness and sadness. For as long as history is, suicide has been traditional, expected in most cultures. We await the day governments cease declaring 'zero suicide' wars and society accepting it as a social and human fact.

Baechler has a nice phrasing of a sad sentiment in his *Suicides*. He says all books on suicide end with recommendations or, rather, exhortations about humankind needing to get rid of such calamities—'but such pieties change not a whit the reality of suicide, no more than the incessant advertisements in newspapers and on radio and television influence the number of highway accidents' (Baechler 1979: 34).

This work seeks to change, even a whit, the conventional thinking about suicide. It offers a much broader understanding of suicide, a wider perspective from the professional health carers, and a more realistic approach to suicide alleviation. Our Western society may well medicalise practically everything, but a dose of philosophy and a touch of sociology can do so much better than antidepressants.

Colin Tatz (Sydney)

Simon Tatz (Melbourne)

June 2019.

References

Baechler, J. (1979). *Suicides*. New York: Basic Books.

Broz, L., & Münster, D. (Eds.). (2016). *Suicide and agency: Anthropological perspectives on self-destruction, personhood, and power*. London: Routledge.

Camus, A. (1955). *The myth of Sisyphus*. London: Hamish Hamilton.

Dilthey, W. (1989). *Introduction to the human sciences*. Princeton, NJ: Princeton University Press.

Douglas, J. (1967). *The social meanings of suicide*. Princeton, NJ: Princeton University Press.

Kaysen, S. (1993). *Girl, interrupted*. New York: Random House.

Lester, D. (1996). *Patterns of suicide and homicide in the world*. New York: Nova Science Publishers, Inc.

Shneidman, E. (1972). Foreword. In A. Cain (Ed.), *Survivors of suicide*. Springfield, IL: Charles C. Thomas Pub Ltd.

Szasz, T. (1998). *Fatal freedom: The ethics and politics of suicide*. Santa Barbara, CA: Praeger Publishers.

Tatz, C. (2005). *Aboriginal suicide is different: A portrait of life and self-destruction*. Canberra: Aboriginal Studies Press.

World Health Organization. (2011). Suicide rates per 100,000 by country, year and sex. (Online).

Chapter 2
The Sound of Suicide

Suicide. A sideways word. A word that people whisper and mutter and cough: a word that must be squeezed out behind cupped palms or murmured behind closed doors. It was only in dreams that I heard the word shouted, screamed.

—Lauren Oliver [American novelist, author of *Before I Fall* (Oliver 2010)]

Taboos, though unadmitted, are potent. What is it that people fear? What they don't understand. The civilised man is not a whit different from the savage in this respect. The new always carries with it the sense of violation, of sacrilege. What is dead is sacred; what is new, that is, different, is evil, dangerous, or subversive.

—Henry Miller [American writer Henry Miller (1891–1980), *The Air-Conditioned Nightmare* (1970)]

Abstract We explore the 'for' and 'against' arguments about suicide; we compare other causes of death and the extraordinary responses to suicide; the frustration of unravelling the causes of suicide; the taboos and stigmas of suicide as shown by the medical examiners' verdicts in the Twin Towers disaster of 9/11.

Keywords Suicide debates · The suicide enigma · 'Falling' vs 'jumping'.

The *hissing* sound of suicide evokes emotions and passion in most Western societies: consternation, discomfort, dismay, exasperation, sorrow and sometimes relief and sympathy. American writer Jennifer Niven noted that people rarely bring flowers to a suicide (Niven 2015). Objectivity and dispassion are not in the vocabulary when it comes to self-destruction.

'You wouldn't call it normal, would you?' is a common rhetorical question, one we have heard from the medical profession. The history books tell us otherwise. Suicide is an ineluctable feature of life in almost all societies. It was first documented in Egypt about two millennia Before the Common Era (BCE). Assisted suicide wasn't

© Springer Nature Switzerland AG 2019
C. Tatz and S. Tatz, *The Sealed Box of Suicide*,
https://doi.org/10.1007/978-3-030-28159-5_2

far behind. As far back as the second century CE, the Greek philosopher Celsus wrote: 'For it is the part of a prudent man first not to touch a case he cannot save and not to risk the appearance of having killed one whose lot is but to die' (Warraich 2017: 232). While suicide is now high on the list of public enemies—alien, alienating, confronting and, above all, affronting—it is still shrouded by taboo. It is to be resisted and prevented, nay, eliminated—so declaim some governments. And assisted suicide is close behind, with only a handful of Western jurisdictions legalising euthanasia, more commonly called assisted dying.

The World Health Organization documents 800,000 suicides annually. Thousands more are classified as 'unknown' cause (see Appendix for the statistics of 41 nations). Suicide is almost three times as common as murder—and would be more common if coronial systems were not so disposed to avoiding suicide verdicts whenever possible. Yet suicide is denounced and deprecated as an affliction, a malediction. It was criminalised and made punishable until recent times in some societies. It is regarded as an outrage in many religions yet honoured in others. But whatever the mood swings in societies across the generations, suicide is standard behaviour. Unacceptable, certainly undesirable to many, yes, but it is a stark social reality.

Given the reactions, and taking account of the taboos that still enshroud suicide, can there be, or should there be, 'sides' to the question? The 'pro'-argument—which is our stance—is that individuals have dominion over their bodies, not the state, not society, and that the taking of that life is—in the phrase of the late psychiatrist Thomas Szasz—'the fatal freedom' (Szasz 1998). Natascha Kampusch—a Viennese girl abducted for eight years from 1988—said of her ordeal that 'suicide seemed to me the greatest kind of freedom, a release from everything, from a life that had been ruined a long time ago' (Kampusch 2010, see Footnote 1).

The body as property, over which ownership or control is or can be vested, is of importance in this age of organ transplants (Johnstone 2007). We discuss this later. We will also look at the views of Holocaust prisoner Jean Améry and his proposition that it is appropriate that people end lives lived in ignominy, in desperate physical or mental pain or in hopelessness. In his opinion, the suicide should not be considered 'the last great outsider' (Améry 1999: xii). Améry is important to us: yes, he killed himself—not amidst death in Auschwitz but some 16 years later amid life. In Chap. 6, we discuss categories of suicide and the importance of differentiating between kinds of suicide (especially for those in prevention work). Améry's suicide illustrates both a genre and a category of suicide. The genre is Baechler's *oblative suicide*, that is, transfigurational in the sense that one state of being, or one life, is exchanged for another, another state called death. The category, shared with the celebrated suicider poet Sylvia Plath, may well be an example of one of the 36 categories we discuss: in these cases, *validation* or *authenticity suicide*.

The 'anti'-perspective has long been basic canon in several major religions, beginning with Judaism and taken up with great vigour by Christianity, certainly from the time of St. Augustine of Hippo (354–430 CE). From him came the doctrine that only God giveth and only God taketh, making it sinful for anyone else to end a life

(Battin 2015: 174–181). Centuries later, the English Catholic cleric and writer G. K. Chesterton (1874–1936) would proclaim that 'not only is suicide a sin, it is *the* sin … It is the ultimate and absolute evil … the refusal to take the oath of loyalty to life' (Chesterton 1908). The 'anti'-side talks about 'wasted life', 'senseless actions', but also about the aftershocks of a suicide: the impacts on the immediate family and circle of friends and on the number of official and professional people who have to deal with the aftermath. In this sense, the suicider's[1] pain has ended, but it has been passed on in a ripple effect to those close to them.

There is also a somewhat conventional view, long held in Europe, that suicide is not only deviant but an assault on the ways people are expected to die, something that contradicts 'the natural instinct' to live (Morrisey 2006: 1). Suicide is seen as an insult and an affront, a crucial matter we address.

We treat the *for* and *against* views. We don't see suicide in the sin sense, but fully accept that many religious persons do. We don't subscribe to the view that suicide is a form of murder or that one suicide inexorably leads to another in a contagious way. Nor do we accept that suicide is always (or mainly) associated with mental illness. And we see little prospect of success in current suicide prevention programmes. Rather, we hope to elicit more concentration on external factors, the contextual elements, the connections and lost connections that operate in so many suicides. A major dilemma, certainly, but our inclination is to regard the suicider's right to end their pain as more important than the repercussions for the living. Why is the grief at loss of a loved one by suicide viewed, or felt often enough, as a greater grief than a loss by cancer?

Yet another dilemma faces us: is not the whole framework of today's suicide a false or at least an artificial construct that has resulted in disproportionate responses? Given the role and place of suicide in human history, and given that suicide is not some alien attack on our society or an 'epidemic' within it, why do we have such emotional (and financial) investment in strategies to prevent it? There are other causes of death of similar number that do not attract anything like the reactions to suicide, nothing like the money raised for prevention and awareness. We argue that in most Western societies suicide is more affronting than confronting.

Nobody knows for certain why people kill themselves (Bering 2018; Lester 1987, 1988, 1989, 1996). If we did, we'd be able to address what Western society deems a serious, if not a momentous, problem. We have before us a remarkable book by two former Metropolitan Life Insurance Company (New York) statisticians, Louis Dublin and Bessie Bunzel. Written in 1933, and with an enormous database to hand, they concluded that 'there is no single factor responsible for suicide':

---

[1] Correct grammar indicates that a person who takes their life is a 'suicide'. To distinguish the verb from the noun, we have used 'suicider' rather than 'a suicide' for such a person.

even when some one cause would seem to dominate the picture, closer investigation discovers that it never stands in isolation but is bound up with various other considerations lying hidden or confused below the surface. (Dublin and Bunzel 1933: 14).[2]

Jennifer Michael Hecht's *Stay* is an admirable analysis of suicide across the ages, and she exercises her right and judgment to come out against the behaviour. But she is inappropriately generalising when she asserted that suicide 'is the tragic end result of depression' (Hecht 2013: 18). In some circumstances, suicide makes sense, as when a person or a group faces impossible choices, as discussed fully in Chap. 7. We show just how many bases there are for suicides in different cultures and eras, none of which have any relationship to or origins in 'depression'. Most often society engages in a form of syllogism: since we can't explain why people take their lives, the reason they do so must lie beyond reasoned explanation and thus resides in the realm of the surreal, the irrational, in the 'disturbed mind'. There is now good reason from research to question the common 'truth' that 90% of all suicides are caused by mental illness (Hjelmeland and Knizer 2017; Shahtahmasebi 2013).

Margaret Pabst Battin's superlative volume—*The Ethics of Suicide* (2015)—takes us on a global suicide journey from Egyptian Didactic Tales some 2050 years Before the Common Era (BCE), to the Hebrew Bible, to Homer, Thomas Aquinas in the thirteenth century, to Martin Luther, John Donne, Voltaire, David Hume, Georg Hegel, Sigmund Freud and to the present. From early scripture lessons, one recalls a vengeful Samson who, with rational premeditation, brought the temple of the Philistines down upon himself in about 1078 BCE; that some 25 years later King Saul wittingly chose to fall upon his sword rather than be run through by an uncircumcised enemy; that at the death of Jesus, the apostle Judas hanged himself.[3] Ahitophel was a supporter of Absalom, King David's third son, who revolted against his father. He, too, went home, set his house in order, and hanged himself (*2 Samuel* 17:23). And, memorably, in about 30 BCE, Cleopatra knowingly clutched a venomous asp to her bosom. [The remarkable English metaphysical poet John Donne (1572–1631) treated these biblical suicides in his famous *Biathanatos* (published in 1608)]. Neither biblical testament discussed suicide, neither condemned it, and neither had a word for self-death other than to describe the act, as in 'Judas hanged himself'.

Historically, suicide has been applauded, then outlawed, excoriated and punished. It has been posited as the only truly philosophical problem (Camus 1955). It has been explained as the ultimate refuge for those who find life not worth living, and it has been hailed as mankind's final or 'fatal freedom'. To the question 'what counts as suicide?, a younger American philosopher Peter Windt answered: 'not so easy to say' (Windt in Battin 2015: 711–716). In Chap. 6, we categorise the several genres of suicide and the many forms or types of self-cessation, some 36 that we know of. Yes, suicide is suicide, but many suicides are very different in motive, nature, form,

---

[2]Many life insurance policies were void if the insured suicided or suicided within one year of taking out a policy. Insurance 'detectives' like Dublin and Bunzel would have been the most painstaking of all death investigators.

[3]*Judges* 16:30 for Samson; *1 Samuel* 31:4 for Saul; *Matthew* 27:5 for Judas.

context, in 'the conditions hidden and confused below the surface' (Dublin and Bunzel 1933; Durkheim 2013 edn). We discuss the failure of prevention strategies to distinguish these differences—akin to asking medical professionals to treat some hundred forms of cancer as if it were one affliction.

'Of all the escape mechanisms', the acerbic social critic H. L. Mencken once wrote, 'death is the most efficient' (Mencken 1916). The resort to that mechanism is today widely presented as quintessentially a 'mental health issue', an 'illness' commonly and often dogmatically defined as 'depression', the 'black dog', and a condition 'beyond blue'. Such illness is commonly seen as a consequence of vulnerability to an early traumatic experience such as childhood sexual abuse, misuse of drugs or alcohol, employment history, a broken relationship, and to genetics. On rarer occasion, some official bodies—like Britain's National Health Service (NHS)—added external elements to the list of mental health conditions of schizophrenia, borderline personality disorder, anorexia, bipolar disorder and severe depression (*NHS Choices*, online). The addendum on 'other risk factors for suicide' comes across as if an asterisked, marginal footnote: being a war veteran, an armed forces member, gay, homeless, working close to suicide modes (meaning doctors and pharmacists), or on discharge from prison, or exposure to those who have taken their lives. In 2018, the Australian media brought to light the high number of distressed and self-deceased ambulance officers (especially in New South Wales) who have resorted to stealing Fentanyl[4] vials from their emergency kits to dose themselves and 'overdose' in some cases.

Few people talk about history, the legacies of history, geography, space, access to social institutions, social or racial discrimination and alienation, physical illness or disability (see Critical Response Pilot Report, University of Western Australia 2017). In Chaps. 4 and 7, we talk about history, about those who took their own lives rather than have a tyrannical regime take them, about the barely known misfortunes of African slaves in America who suicided rather than suffer their mistreatment (Snyder 2015) and the South American tribes who killed themselves *en masse* rather than live under Spanish colonial repression (Stannard 1993).

A respected investigative writer talked learnedly about the 'epidemic' of mental illness (Whitaker 2010)—but even epidemics trail history and have a continuing presence. It is rare for anyone to discuss the myth of 'happiness', let alone question the unreality that we have a God-given human right to be happy, that not to enjoy that status on a permanent basis is both an aberration and a symptom of unwellness.

No one knows with certainty how many people suicide. The world-wide estimate is that each year between 800,000 and one million people wilfully end their lives. The data may be 'volatile', according to the authors of the 2016 'Causes of Death' report (Richie and Roser 2016), but 817,148 persons ended their lives in 2016. That represents 1.49% of all deaths. As discussed later, this figure is an underestimation—because coroners and medical examiners are reluctant to determine suicide in less

---

[4] A strong opioid used for pain.

than obvious cases, because more such officials have been inconsistent on levels of proof required, because of the often vigorous family resistance to a finding of suicide and because of the black cloud of suicide stigma that hovers over many societies. In perspective, the latest data world-wide (2016) show road toll deaths were 1.34 million, liver disease accounted for 1.26 million deaths, tuberculosis 1.21 million, HIV/AIDS 1.03 million, malaria 719,000, homicide 390,794, drug disorders 143,775 and terrorism deaths estimated at 34,676. These figures may be inexact, and they will change, but they do indicate that suicide is not arithmetically aberrant.

Amid any number of twists and turns, self-destruction has been celebrated, encouraged, deemed a badge of honour or martyrdom, branded as cowardice, condemned as a sin and a blasphemy, decreed as criminal, softened by euphemism as something other than it is and is today lamented as a calamity, 'a tragic event'.

Joseph Zubin (1900–1990), the renowned American psychopathologist and expert on schizophrenia, concluded that 'in most behavioural disorders, we have at least part of the process at hand for examination', but 'in suicide, all we usually have is the end result, arrived at by a variety of paths'. 'Unravelling the cause after the fact', he declared, 'is well-nigh impossible' (quoted in Alvarez 1974, Penguin edition).

There can be no clearer example of the 'well-nigh impossible' unravelling of intention than the 9/11 catastrophe that resulted from the al-Qaeda destruction of the Twin Towers buildings in New York City in 2001. Judgment of the fate of some 200 who jumped to certain death will long be a quest and a debate. The Twin Towers disaster also revealed the strength of the taboos and the denialism that suffuse suicide, even in medical examiners' courts.

Some 3,000 people died in the 9/11 inferno, but the enduring image, *the* haunting image, is the iconic photograph captured by Richard Drew that became known as the 'falling man'. Were the falling individuals suiciders? They faced a Hobson's choice, no choice at all as between incineration and death from a height. But the very notion of suicide caused immense distress. It divided families and those whose business is the study and prevention of suicide.

The US Centers for Disease Control and Prevention (CDC), under their Operational Criteria for Determination of Suicide, classify a death as a suicide if a medical examiner[5] can establish that the death is both self-inflicted and intentional (Timmermans 2005). Dr. Charles Hirsch, the forensic pathologist and chief medical examiner of New York City who oversaw the identification of 9/11 victims, didn't believe the 'falling' persons were suicides. He found all deaths to be homicides. Although some of the 'jumpers' made a decision to end their lives prematurely, their deaths were not considered to be self-inflicted, voluntary or intentional acts. The term used by the medical examiner was 'fallers', clearly indicating that they fell—unusually, unintentionally or accidentally—rather than that they took a conscious decision to jump.

---

[5]In the USA, medical examiners are often trained forensic pathologists. They list cause of death into five categories: natural, accident, homicide, suicide and undetermined.

Margaret Battin asked us *not* to consider the 9/11 jumpers as a form of mass, and very public, suicide. Her considered view was that suicide can be defined by the purpose behind the death:

> … think of the 9/11 jumpers in this way – do we stress the mechanism of their deaths or the perfectly understandable, reasonable intentions they had in escaping a much worse death by incineration? … To ask whether the 9/11 jumpers were suicides is to trade on the very negative connotations associated with the term suicide and to imply that they did something wrong or perhaps even sinful. (McDermott 2017)

Suicide scholar David Lester explained that some family members disavowed the notion that their relative jumped, 'saying that jumping would have been a betrayal' (Lester 2013). Presumably, these family members meant a betrayal of every custom and norm society holds about suicide: it is sinful, shameful, stigmatising, an act of cowardice. Such was the extreme reaction to the notion that some of those who jumped/fell could even be considered suicides that when, one year after 9/11, an exhibition at New York's Rockefeller Centre featured a bronze sculpture called *Tumbling Woman* it was closed within a week amid protests and bomb threats.

So why yet another book to add to the laden libraries of learned journals, treatises and books on the suicide enigma? The short answer is that in order to *prevent* suicide—or to use less pretentious terms, to deflect or alleviate or mitigate self-harm, especially among the young—we have to look at all likely causal factors and contexts and not blindly follow the biomedical model that has tried, in the words of the English literary critic Alfred Alvarez, to 'remove [suicide] from the vulnerable, volatile world of human beings and hidden [it] safely away in the isolation wards of science' (Alvarez 1974: 92–93, Penguin edition). Since his remarkable book, *The Savage God*, a new debate and a new genre of writing have emerged on 'epidemics' of mental illness and the value, or not, of 'doctoring the mind' (Bentall 2009). Alvarez would have admired (as we do) much of the writing of the Hungarian-American psychiatrist Thomas Szasz (1920–2012). Several of his book titles are memorable: *The Theology of Medicine* (1979), *The Myth of Mental Illness* (1972), *The Manufacture of Madness* (1997). Our framework, like that of anthropologist Marx (1976), is that suicide is an act of violence that arises out of the social order, and it can only *begin* to be explained (and understood) in a social rather than a medical context. Almost a hundred years earlier, Enrico (Henry) Morselli, the Italian psychiatrist, explained the high rates of Italian suicide: in times of cultural and economic fragmentation, when nations were struggling to be born, suicide escalated (Morselli 1882). So, too, in Lithuania and Latvia in the 1990s. The social order arising out of disorder explains much about human behaviour.

The biomedical model dominates. It contends that illness and disease are located solely within the individual and that treatment is predominantly, if not exclusively, surgical, psychotherapeutic and/or pharmacological. Such a lens and such a location exonerate society from any responsibility in the aetiology of the disease. Biomedicine de-socialises and de-contextualises disease and explains *any* social phenomena, where on the rare occasions, they are considered relevant, in medical terms. The patient, not society or anything arising out of society, is the ultimate repository of responsibility (Filc 2004: 1276–1279). Szasz once described this universe as 'the medicalisation of everything'.

There is no one '–ology' that has mastered suicide causality, let alone prevention in the broad sense. If we are to make better sense of suicide and the approaches to it, we argue that there is more to learn from philosophy than any other discipline. If the great thinker Benjamin Franklin (1706–1790) was right, then nine out of ten persons are would-be suicides. That leaves us with an indelible existential problem, hardly a medical one. Suicide is not a Siamese twin of mental illness in all or even in most instances. There is no certitude that the suicide idea is, somehow, a diagnosable and treatable medical condition—not just a patient's symptom of melancholic or unhappy feelings. There is also no shortage of proclamations and mission statements that the phenomenon can be both 'solved' and prevented. Assuming that one day science will find that elusive depression gene,[6] or the even more elusive suicide gene, or the hitherto undetectable chemical that causes 'imbalance' in the brain, what then? Surely not implanted beepers that will signal the propensity of teenagers to want to end lives almost before they have begun? And if the beepers were to beep, what then?

Western society is investing fair sums of money in prevention strategies, by way of government funding and by private sponsorships and bequests. There is not much evidence of their efficacy, whether suicide rates decrease long-term as a result of their programmes. The evidence is stark: the rates are not decreasing in any uniform ways that suggest prevention approaches are achieving universal changes in suicide numbers.[7] There is the added problem that prevention agencies don't appear to differentiate between the 36 categories of suicide we present, and many of them simply cannot be approached in the same or even in a similar way.

Before we discuss that issue, some fundamental questions need to be asked. Why are we so fixated on addressing this particular problem? Why is it a problem, or one any more so than drug and alcohol abuse? We are saddened, often sickened, yet accepting that people become addicted, ruin their lives and those of their families, drive recklessly and engage in risky behaviour. But we are not only confronted but seemingly even more *affronted* and threatened by suicide, and we need to question this response.

The premeditated cutting short of a life that will end in abject and untreatable pain also sits outside the suicide paradigm. Often enough doctors ensure the 'quiet deaths' of the terminally ill, either by an act of commission or omission. Many societies accept (or at the very least, rarely investigate) a life terminated before the cancer renders the last weeks of life an excruciatingly painful suffering to witness. Suicide 'preventionists' recognise voluntary euthanasia as understandable, even reasonable,

---

[6] On 14 May 2019, the *Sydney Morning Herald* reported that the QIMR Berghofer Medical Research Institute in Queensland had identified 31 genes as at-risk factors in depression.

[7] In the USA, for example, suicide rates have increased in almost every state between 1999 and 2016, as reported in *Vital Signs*, 7 June 2018.

just as they recognise that leaping from a burning inferno is probably not a suicide per se. For Armenians in Turkey, Jews in Nazi Europe, young Syrian girls, for those sufferers of chronic pain that resists all palliative care or the soon-to-be incinerated Tower victims—these suicides are not caused by mental illness, prescription medication, lack of biomedical interventions, psychiatry services or shortage of suicide crisis hotlines.

We call this book *The Sealed Box* because we wish to open up to question many aspects of suicide, including the data sets and statistical empires that influence health care, funding and media coverage. Suicide is under-reported. The prevention strategies and methodologies are under-evaluated. It is not even transparent what is meant by suicide prevention: whose agency over their own lives are we trying to prevent, and why? The big question here is why there is so much effort, so much clamour, to stop people from having control over their lives—and their manner of death.

Suicide prevention is about the living. Suicides most often leave behind grief, destruction of families and friends and enduring pain of loss. The questions are almost always: why did they do it? why didn't I see it coming? what could I have done to stop it? For others, it is anger and blame at the 'system' and agencies that 'failed'. There must be a reason, an explanation, a cause, a condition or disorder. They should have seen it; and if not, blame is apportioned: not enough investment in mental health services; not enough crisis lines; they haven't eliminated stigma; media coverage encourages copycat suicides; we must reach out and 'start a conversation' and ask if everyone is 'okay'; if only there was more money, more apps, more websites and interventions. If only …

At some point in modern times, suicide became a medical matter. Doctors—of the mind and body—became the authorities on suicidal behaviour. Suicide was declared a problem primarily of the mind, the mentally unwell, the depressed and the deranged. Suicide, say some medical professionals, may be caused by a gene that medical science can eventually locate and treat. Suicide has become a race to pinpoint the diagnoses and the antidote. It is an approach that isn't working. Raw data tell us that Australian suicide rates fell from 17.5 per 100,000 in 1963 to 11.8 in 2016 and then rose in 2017 to 12.7. This may be due to changes in methodology with new coronial reporting procedures showing an increase in rates or factors beyond the data sets. In sum, the millions invested in 'prevention' warrant rigorous evaluation—for example, to reveal how much is devoted to bereavement, how much to prevention as such.

Suicide prevention—'preventionists' as we call them—has its own chapter here, one likely to cause some consternation among the many organisations funded to forestall intentional death. Suicide prevention is something of a furphy [an Australian term for an erroneous or improbable story]. Suicides are not being 'prevented' in the manner of polio or smallpox. (At best, 'prevention' means efforts to educate persons to alternative choices.) As with illicit drug use, the preventionists are not winning the war against suicide, a fruitless battle if history has any meaning. At best, as we will examine, there are some ways to deflect and postpone a few categories of intended suicide, but only a few, perhaps 5 of the 36 categories we discuss, or 14%. Many forms of the behaviour are indirect; that is, there are no overt physical or outward symptoms that attract attention. Several categories are deeply internalised, rarely susceptible to any articulation to a therapist. Some categories can be mitigated, stayed, and possibly even contained to some degree, but generally, it can't be diagnosed, treated, and prevented in the innoculatory sense of the word. Only those with a history of attempts can be monitored and assisted; even so, we have no way of knowing how many of that group do or don't go on to complete their goal.

Suicide Prevention Australia (SPA), the major organisation in this country, has proposed a statute for a federal office of suicide prevention and a federal minister of suicide prevention as a way of stopping the phenomenon.[8] Such is the nature of desperation.

References

Alvarez, A. (1974). *The savage god: A study of suicide*. London: Penguin Books.

Améry, J. (1999). *On suicide: A discourse on voluntary death*. Bloomington, IN: Indiana University Press.

Battin, M. P. (2015). *The ethics of suicide: Historical sources*. Oxford: Oxford University Press.

Bentall, R. (2009). *Doctoring the mind: Why psychiatric treatments fail*. London: Penguin Books.

Bering, J. (2018). *Suicidal: Why we kill ourselves*. Chicago: Chicago University Press.

Camus, A. ([1955] 1991). *The myth of Sisyphus and other essays*. New York: Vintage International.

Chesterton, G. K. ([1908] 2009 edn). *Orthodoxy*. Chicago: Moody Press.

Donne, J. ([1608] 1982). In M. Rudick & M. P. Battin (Eds.), *Biathanatos* (a modern spelling edition). New York: Garland Publishing Inc.

Dublin, L. & Bunzel, B. (1933). *To be or not to be: A study in suicide*. New York: Harrison Smith and Robert Haas.

Durkheim, É. ([1897] 2013). *Suicide: A study in sociology*. New York: The Free Press.

Filc, D. (2004). The medical text: Between biomedicine and hegemony. *Social Science and Medicine, 59,* 1276–1279.

Hecht, J. M. (2013). *Stay: A history of suicide and the philosophies against it*. New Haven CT: Yale University Press.

Hjelmeland, H., & Knizer, B. (2017). Suicide and mental disorders: A discourse of politics, power, and vested interests. *Death Studies*. https://doi.org/10.1080/07481187.2017.1332905.

Johnstone, R. (2007). *Crossing the human/animal divide: Rethinking legal personhood in the context of animal to human transplants*, Ph.D. thesis, University of Sydney.

Kampusch, N. (2010). *3,096 days in captivity*. London: Penguin Books.

Lester, D. (1987). *Suicide as a learned behavior*. Springfield, IL: Charles Thomas.

Lester, D. (1988). *Suicide from a psychological perspective*. Springfield IL: Charles Thomas.

Lester, D. (1989). *Suicide from a sociological perspective*. Springfield IL: Charles Thomas.

Lester, D. (1996). *Patterns of suicide and homicide in the world*. New York: Nova Science Publishers Inc.

---

[8] *Hobart Mercury,* 16 May 2019.

Lester, D. (2013). Those who jumped from the Twin Towers on 9/11: Suicides or not? Richard Stockton College, USA. *Suicidology Online 2013, 4*, 117–121. http://www.suicidology-online.com/pdf/SOL-2013-4-117-121.pdf.

Marx, E. (1976). *The social context of violent behaviour: A Social study of an Israeli immigrant town*. London: Routledge & Kegan Paul.

McDermott, M. (2017, September 11). Redefining 9/11 jumpers. *Utah Daily Chronicle*. http://dailyutahchronicle.com/2017/09/11/jumpers/.

Mencken, H. L. ([1916] 2010 edn). *Book of burlesques*. New York: Valdebooks.

Miller, H. (1970). *The air-conditioned nightmare*. New York: New Directions Books.

Morrissey, S. (2006). *Suicide and the body politic in imperial Russia*. Cambridge: Cambridge University Press.

Morselli, E. (Henry). (1882). *Suicide: An essay on comparative moral statistics*. New York: D. Appleton and Company.

Niven, J. (2015). *All the bright places*. New York: Alfred Knopf.

Oliver, L. (2010). *Before I fall*. New York: HarperCollins.

Report of the Critical Response Pilot Project. (2017). *Aboriginal and Torres Strait Islander Suicide prevention evaluation project* (Pat Dudgeon, Jill Milroy, Yvonne Luxford and Christopher Holland).

Richie, H., & Roser, M. (2016). *Causes of death*. Our World of Data. https://ourworldindata.org/causes-of-death.

Shahtahmasebi, S. (2013). Examining the claim that 80–90% of suicide cases had depression. *Front Public Health, 1*(62).

Snyder, T. (2015). *The power to die: Slavery and suicide in British North America*. Chicago: Chicago University Press.

Stannard, D. (1993). *American holocaust: The conquest of the new world*. London: Oxford University Press.

Szasz, T. (1972). *The myth of mental illness*. London: Paladin.

Szasz, T. (1979). *The theology of medicine: The political-philosophic foundations of medical ethics*. Syracuse, NY: Syracuse University Press.

Szasz, T. (1997). *The manufacture of madness: A comparative study of the inquisition and the mental health movement*. Syracuse, NY: Syracuse University Press.

Szasz, T. (1998). *Fatal freedom: The ethics and politics of suicide*. Santa Barbara, CA: Praeger Publishers.

Timmermans, S. (2005, April). Suicide determination and the professional authority of medical examiners. *American Sociological Review, 70*(2), 311–333. Published by: American Sociological Association Stable. http://www.jstor.org/stable/4145372.

Warraich, H. (2017). *Modern death: How medicine changed the end of life*. London: Duckworth Overlook.

Whitaker, R. (2010). *Anatomy of an epidemic: Magic bullets, psychiatric drugs and the astonishing rise of mental illness*. New York: Broadway Books above.

Chapter 3
Depressing Thoughts

... and, for many a time I have been half in love with easeful Death, ... Now more than ever seems it rich to die, To cease upon the midnight with no pain

—John Keats: 'Ode to a Nightingale' (1819)

To die—to sleep, No more; and by a sleep to say we end The heart-ache and the thousand natural shocks That flesh is heir to, 'tis a consummation Devoutly to be wish'd.

—Shakespeare: *Hamlet*, Act III, Scene 1

Abstract The fascination of suicide; fads and fashions in psychiatry; the *Diagnostic and Statistical Manual of Mental Disorder (DSM)* and its influence on society; the dominion and dominance of the biomedical model of suicide and mental illness; an introduction to critical suicide studies and its agendas.

Keywords Medical fashions · The *DSM* 'bible' · The normality of distress

To be or not to be? Hamlet's conundrum says it all: the wish to end the heartache and all the other shocks that befall humankind. 'To die, to sleep' and perchance to dream (of better things). And an extraordinary ode by Keats, one given to much speculation. Some say it is an address to ecstasy; others discern a dawning of impermanence, of mortality. Perhaps a tribute to wine: 'a beaker full of the warm South, /with beaded bubbles winking at the brim'—and, certainly, a salute to the oblivion wrought by 'a draught of vintage'. That he was on his way to dying of pulmonary tuberculosis (in 1821, aged 25) no doubt propelled the poem. But the words quoted here are plain enough: suicide, or at least what the professional jargon calls 'suicide ideation'. How else does one explain the need to get away from 'The weariness, the fever, and the fret', the contention that it 'is rich to die' and, best of all, to 'cease upon the midnight with no pain'? We can as readily conjecture that his massive lung haemorrhages would have made an exit from life—and an entrance to a state of death—'easeful'.

'Man's ability to kill himself has been a source of fascination since the beginning of human society. Philosophers from Marcus Aurelius and Seneca to Camus … have contributed voluminously to its study'—the words of Norman Kreitman (1927–2012), a British academic psychiatrist who coined the term *parasuicide* for those who attempt the act (Kreitman 1987: 758–760). Writing the entry on suicide for the *Oxford Companion to the Mind*, Kreitman contended that 'rational suicide is exceedingly rare, if indeed it exists at all' (in Gregory 1987: 759). Exalted thinkers like Baruch Spinoza (1632–1677) and Immanuel Kant (1724–1804) were concerned about the self and wrote a great deal about rational suicide, which does indeed exist (as we discuss in later chapters). Suicide today is steadfastly characterised as irrational, yet the innovative statute on assisted death, enacted by Australia's state of Victoria in 2017,[1] demands that one criterion to legitimise the action is that the person requesting such death must have 'decision-making capacity' (thus excluding those with mental illness). In many cultures, suicide is a noble and honourable way out of a dilemma. So which is it: rational actions or minds so disturbed that they don't know what they're doing, people incapable of handling or controlling their own agency?

Philosophers were not just writers on self-destruction but were often enough the sentinels of suicide in society. Certainly, the priests were once the guardians, followed by the lawyers who were intent on protecting a suicider's assets from compulsory forfeiture to the Crown, a normal practice until the mid-nineteenth century. The task of dealing with suicide then fell to the biomedical world and it is likely to be cemented there for decades to come. In that model, suicide is confined to a complication of mental illness, usually depression—regardless of geographic, historic, political and social contexts—factors critical, for example, in Armenian, Jewish, Japanese, Hindu, Australian Aboriginal, Māori, Amerindian and Inuit suicide.

The restricted zone of a medicalised suicide is now under serious challenge. Critical suicide studies—a new movement—has much in common with what is now called critical medical anthropology. In their way, both sub-disciplines have moved away from a preoccupation with micro-studies, away from a narrow focus on tissue samples, body substances and biological disorders generally. These areas of study are not in search of a middle ground but another ground. They analyse the socio-economic forces and power differences that influence access to health care and deal with intervention, prevention and policy issues. They have evolved because of the way in which the traditional medical model has stared itself blind looking for the source of malfunction in the individual and never, or hardly ever, looking at cultural and socio-economic factors, still less in historical, social and political contexts. Later, we discuss suicide among the Armenian and the Jewish victims of genocide in the last century, and the Lithuanian rates of suicide following the end of Soviet hegemony in 1990. Those contexts were avowedly political, not medical.

---

[1] *The Voluntary Assisted Dying Act 2017* (Victoria).

Critical suicide scholars are in search of a much broader agency (White et al. 2016). They look at *suicide in context* and not merely inside the heads of the parasuicides and of those deceased. The new movement is addressing the 'science' of suicide, the social significance of suicide, the contextual or external factors and the coronial reporting problems. It also proposes a sensible rethinking of attitudes towards, and education about, this taboo-laden topic. Those trained in the arts, humanities and social sciences are now addressing a subject hitherto secreted in the cloistered world of the medical and allied professions since the start of the twentieth century.[2]

Mental illness is a quagmire. In his book, *Shrinks*, Jeffrey Lieberman, professor of psychiatry at Columbia University and director of the New York State Psychiatric Institute, has an eloquent chapter on what he calls 'A Farrago of Diagnoses' (Lieberman 2015: 87–116). He quoted writer Rita Mae Brown: 'The statistics on sanity are that one out of every four Americans is suffering from some form of mental illness. Think of your three best friends. If they're okay, then it's you'. Arguments rage about whether it is a sickness of the 'mind', the 'self', the soul, the biological brain or of society.

Psychiatry was the name given to the new discipline by the German physician and anatomist Johann Reil in 1808. He perceived it as the medicine or the healing of the soul. [The Afrikaans language of South Africa translates the word as *sielkunde*, meaning psychology or study of the soul.] It is a field of thought and therapy which has yet to find the essence of the 'illness' that it seeks to heal, that which we call suicide, defined in 1755 by the lexicographer Samuel Johnson in his great *Dictionary of the English Language* as: 'self-murder; the horrid crime of destroying one's self'. It was to remain a crime in the Western world's statute books for almost another two centuries. (The UK abolished attempted suicide as a crime in 1961, and India did so in 2017; Australian jurisdictions abolished the offence between 1957 and 1996.) The 'horrid' stigma remains. Some 216 years after Johnson, Alfred (Al) Alvarez, a noted British literary figure, wrote a powerful work on suicide, *The Savage God*, in which he expressed a more enlightened definition: 'suicide is an act of choice, the terms of which are entirely of this world: a man dies by his own hand because he thinks the life he has [is] not worth living' (Alvarez 1974: 74). In the same decade, American scholar Louis Wekstein stated that suicide 'has a mystique and fascination in its sibilants … it is the human act of self-inflicted, self-intentioned cessation' (Wekstein 1979: 27–30).

Psychiatry has undergone waves of change since the days of Johann Riel. The innovations and theories of Sigmund Freud, Alfred Adler and Carl Jung, among others, have had a profound influence on the betterment of lives for more than a century. New schools of thought, dogmas and best practices have come and gone, and still arrive and depart—often enough without regret, apology or the merest hint of chagrin for what was later shown to be insistent, dogmatic misbelief. Theoretical paroxysms have beset the literature on the very nature of mental illness and whether

---

[2]https://criticalsuicidology.net/papers-on-critical-suicidology/.

mental illness resides in brain tissues, in the dysfunction of synapses and other electrical circuits; in the 'head' or 'mind' or in the 'soul' as the very sources of being; in the 'race' that defines one as 'different', deficient, dangerous and undesirable; in the heritable genes, in the elusive suicide gene and the depression gene; in moral and societal deficits; in something called 'orgone'—a hidden form of energy uniting all of nature's elements—the substance of the impeccably credentialed and revered Austrian-American Wilhelm Reich (1897–1957) and which landed him in jail (where he died); in the fraudulent 'animal magnetism' of the once celebrated German Franz Mesmer (1734–1815); and in the latest proposition from the widely touted Daniel Amen—whom the *Washington Post* has described as 'beyond question the most popular psychiatrist in America'. He claimed he can detect mental illness from brain scans, a 'science' more in common with skull-bump phrenology, according to Jeffrey Lieberman (Lieberman 2015; see also Szasz 1997, 1998). Lieberman has written eloquently on the 'untold story of psychiatry': on the fads, fashions, frauds, and finally, on the arrival of what he calls the 'good' psychiatry. Yet in his book's index you will find only two words under the entry for suicide—'*see depression*'.

Lieberman could well have taken a page or two from *Erewhon*, an 1872 satirical work by the English novelist Samuel Butler, an admirer of Darwin's theories. *Erewhon* (seemingly an anagram of nowhere) was a utopian society [possibly set in New Zealand, where he had shorn sheep] in which, among other things, offenders were treated as ill and the ill were perceived as criminals—hence their need of 'straighteners' to iron out what was so obviously out of kilter (Butler 1872, Chap. 10):

> I will give a few examples of the way in which what we should call misfortune, hardship, or disease are dealt with by the Erewhonians, but for the moment will return to their treatment of cases that with us are criminal. As I have already said, these, though not judicially punishable, are recognised as requiring correction. Accordingly, there exists a class of men trained in soul craft, whom they call straighteners, as nearly as I can translate a word which literally means 'one who bends back the crooked'. These men practise much as medical men in England, and receive a quasi surreptitious fee on every visit. They are treated with the same unreserve, and obeyed as readily, as our own doctors — that is to say, on the whole sufficiently — because people know that it is their interest to get well as soon as they can, and that they will not be scouted as they would be if their bodies were out of order, even though they may have to undergo a very painful course of treatment.

Reading Butler, the remarkable psychiatrist Thomas Szasz, Lieberman and then Richard Bentall's *Doctoring the Mind* (2009), one has to ponder seriously, and then question, several aspects of the nature of 'soul-craft', of 'bending back the crooked'. Quite clearly, there are successful treatments and positive outcomes from the ministrations of well-trained professionals. But is all psychiatry 'good psychiatry'?

The *Diagnostic and Statistical Manual of Mental Disorders, Fifth Edition* (called 'DSM-5' for short) is produced by the American Psychiatry Association. This tome has become 'the bible of psychiatry', one that exercises an unparalleled influence on Western society. It has been much criticised, particularly by non-Americans, for telling us—amid the truly serious and sometimes verifiable illnesses and longish lists of psychoses—that you have a 'mathematical deficit disorder' if you can't do arithmetic; that you have a 'communications disorder' if you wave your hands and point too much; that you have a 'substance use disorder' if you smoke cigarettes or gag for your morning coffee; and you have a 'social phobia' if you are shy. An 'adjustment deficit disorder' is where a stressor causes a great deal of stress in one's life—'like a wedding or buying a new home'. It also tells us that more than a dozen disorders are at the base of suicide by children under 14 (see our Chap. 13).

The American Psychiatric Association and much of Western psychiatry in general would have us accept that the world at large is drowning in disorders or Szasz's 'problems in living' and in need of Butler's 'straightening'. It was only in 1973 that that Association voted to undefine homosexuality as a mental disorder (Burton 2015). We live in a Western world populated by a large sector of the 'worried well' who are seduced (or induced) into believing that they are entitled to be "weller" than well.

Another message that comes across, intentionally or not, is that there are no limits to the imperialism and hegemony of the profession that wants to heal the totality of the soul, and a planet of people beset by 'disorder'. In the 1950s, a group of analysts, led by the American William Menninger, issued a manifesto on 'The Social Responsibility of Psychiatry', proclaiming the profession's (quixotic) politico-medical activism against war, poverty and racism (Lieberman 2015: 84). Noteworthy is that the same Samuel Butler later wrote *The Way of All Flesh*, which the Modern Library (the renowned publisher of classics) rates as the twelfth best novel in the English language. It is an apt enough title for the world of limitless disorders, the dispensing of billions of prescription drugs and therapies for which the fees are neither quasi nor surreptitious. Thomas Szasz titled one of his last books *The Medicalization of Everyday Life* (2007).

Is there good psychiatry and good psychology to be found in 'biopower', sometimes called 'biopolitics', terms coined by the eminent French scholar Michel Foucault in 1976 (Foucault 2003)?

> By this I mean a number of phenomena that seem to me to be quite significant, namely, the set of mechanisms through which the basic biological features of the human species became the objects of a political strategy, of a general strategy of power, or, in other words, how, starting from the 18th century, modern Western societies took on board the fundamental biological fact that human beings are a species. This is what I have called biopower.

In short, Foucault's expressions mean government or state control, often enough through coercive power, of individual or population biology. In the Australian state of Tasmania in the 1920s, there were strong proponents of both hereditarian and environment eugenics, each branch seeking ways to control the presence and future of the 'feeble-minded'. This led to the *Mental Deficiency Act* of 1920, the model for other states (Rodwell 1998). The Nazi regime is the foremost example of biopower, one which demonstrated that they could not only control the creation of life but build dedicated facilities for the manufacture of death (Robertson et al. 2017). In the Nazi worldview, the superior 'Aryan race' could not only rival but could even displace God.

Democratic states are capable of exercising biopolitical power. Between 1890 and the 1920s, 30 American states engaged in widespread sterilisation programs, legislated for in statutes with titles like 'Racial Integrity Act(s)'[3]—aimed at fulfilling eugenicist fantasies of eliminating the halt, blind, deaf and the 'feeble-minded'. Two Canadian provinces—Alberta and British Columbia—as well as Czechoslovakia, Sweden, Japan and Switzerland did much the same thing. In a later chapter, we discuss the nature of biopower over Australian Aboriginal lives, beginning (in Foucault's sense) in 1804, gaining momentum in 1897 and continuing to this day (Tatz 2017, Chaps. 6, 7 and 8).

Biopower is not always a malign force: we have epidemiological surveillance systems seeking out sources of epidemics and pandemics, of contagion and contamination, and public health infrastructures. We have seen enough of states defining worthy and unworthy lives, one-child policies as in Taiwan and China, Aboriginal child removal policies in Australia and Canada, Romani ('Gypsy') 'relocations', child removals and sterilisations in Western and Eastern Europe. Many religions and theocratic states exert biopolitical power over their adherents—on sexual mores, marriageability, abortion, contraception, on circumcision of both genders, suicide and where such self-deceased can be buried. The whole suicide controversy is redolent of biopower (Marsh 2010): the state, not the individual, determined who had sovereignty over the living body, prosecuting and hounding those who thought their bodies belonged to them. They are now as determined to prevent what Szasz has called 'the fatal freedom', the final [human rights] freedom. He stated that medical science truly believes that 'anyone who would want to leave [such a healthy and happy] life prematurely must be mad—or bad … In either case, he must be prevented from doing so' (Szasz 1974: 85). Alvarez reminds us of the aphorism coined by the late English philosopher C. E. M. Joad (1891–1953): 'that in England [until the middle of the twentieth century] you must not commit suicide, on pain of being regarded as a criminal if you fail and a lunatic if you succeed' (Alvarez 1974: 66).

Yet another message, spawned by the advertising moguls of Madison Avenue and the dream factories of Hollywood, is that 'happiness' is an inherent and normal state—and a fundamental human right. Philip Wylie, an overlooked American social critic, called it 'A Specific American Myth', a 'bastard legend', namely, the Cinderella story (Wylie 1942: 46–55). The destiny of the kitchen drudge is that a well-to-do handsome male will elevate her from cruel serfdom, pain and unhappiness to a fairy-lit penthouse with a lifetime guarantee of saunas, bliss and rapture. American it may have been, but the 'to-live-is-to-be-happy' legend has made its way fully into the cultural psyches of all Western peoples.

---

[3]One can readily access online the notorious case of Carrie Buck, compulsorily sterilised under the state of Virginia's *Racial Integrity Act* of 1924. She was sterilised as feeble-minded, despite her school grades showing that she wasn't.

The American Declaration of Independence of 1776 laid down the '
right' to 'life, liberty and the pursuit of happiness'. The Irish Proclamati
1916 sought independence for a people determined 'to pursue the h;
prosperity of the whole nation'. Even the solemn hymn to the British Quᴄᴄ..
we 'send her victorious, happy and glorious'. The absence or shortage of happiness
is diagnosed as a sign of unwellness, and that, too, must be addressed medically
and therapeutically. The esteemed thinker and psychiatrist, Viktor Frankl, a survivor
of several Nazi camps, always said that pleasure or 'happiness' is a by-product, a
side effect of life, not the essence of life—which, at base, is to suffer. 'Suffering
is an ineradicable part of life … without suffering and death human life cannot
be complete' (Frankl 1984, edn: 88). Existential frustration and existential distress
are neither 'pathological nor pathogenic', 'and by no means mental disease', he
wrote (Frankl 1946: 125). Conventional Buddhists agree with him: the first of their
Four Noble Truths is that life is about suffering, pain and misery. (A glance at
Judeo-Christian societies tells us much more about suffering than about joy and
'happiness'.)

Existential distress is just that. It is often terrible and terrifying—and normal. Sociologist Allan Horwitz and social work specialist Jerome Wakefield have lamented
'the loss of sadness' and exposed the way in which psychiatry has turned normal sorrow into a depressive disorder (Horwitz and Wakefield 2007). When the Twin Towers
complex was attacked on 9/11 (2001), no fewer than 9000 therapists descended on the
Manhattan scene to 'treat' the survivors for post-traumatic stress-syndrome (PTSD).
The *Washington Post* called the belief that PTSD is ubiquitous among survivors 'a
fallacy that some mental health counsellors are perpetuating in the aftermath of this
tragedy'. It was another way to depict survivors as fragile rather than resilient.[4]

In 2017, the New South Wales Police announced the formation of a new special
unit comprising 'seventeen detectives and mental health experts', to focus on preventing terrorist attacks by those 'fixated' by a religious or ideological belief. This
conjunction and near-equation of ideology with mental illness will, we believe, go
nowhere: it understands neither political ideology nor mental disease (or the 'good'
and godly fundamentalism of many Christian sects). Historian Eric Hobsbawm predicted in 1965 that the West could never win out against the Viet Cong guerrillas
because it had no comprehension of their mindset; and that the Goliath great pow-
ers, with a 'touch of omnipotence', couldn't conceive of democracy losing out to
any inferior system—in Vietnam, Afghanistan, Iraq, Libya, Syria or anywhere else
(Hobsbawm 1998: 200). And so too 'terrorist ideologies'.

The biomedical model is now almost wholly about suicide and parasuicide as
depression, caused by what no one knows exactly. The general and generalised rem-
edy is an antidepressant regimen. We seem to live in a world, at least a Western
world, suffused by serotonin reuptake inhibitors (SSRIs), tricyclic antidepressants

---

[4]Solnit (2009: 219) writing on how communities cohere after disaster, quotes a psychologist writing
to the *New York Times*: 'The public should be very concerned about medicalizing what are human
reactions'.

(TCAs) and monoamine oxidase inhibitors (MAOIs). We should be grateful for the abbreviations of the tabs that take away tension and trauma, thoughts about 'easeful death', and which, to use the opening lines of Keats' poem, lead to a state where 'a drowsy numbness pains/My sense, as though of hemlock I had drunk'. Prozac, Zoloft, Aropax and their brothers and sisters do dull or numb or dumb the senses, those extraordinary 'things' we call emotions. But in their listing of side effects, the pharmaceutical industry almost never tells you, or the Federal Drug Administration (FDA), or anyone else that suicide (and on occasion enough, homicide) is a side effect.[5] No one remembers or wants to remember the case of *Winkler v Eli Lilly Company* in Kentucky, concluded in 1996. The Lilly pharma giant manufactures Prozac in 20 mg packaging (for convenience, they claim), four times the recommended daily dose and, as the court evidence showed, they fudged the trials and 'massaged the data' to present a harmless or relatively harmless set of side effects—listing only the usual dizziness, drowsiness, sleep problems, mild nausea and so on. They omitted mention of suicide (Cornwell 1996). Lilly paid off the litigants—the spouses of eight dead and 12 wounded by a printing plant employee who, in 1989, had taken the conveniently packaged Prozac, then walked into the factory and sprayed all he could see with an AK assault rifle (and then suicided). Lilly paid undisclosed sums to the litigants in a secret deal. 'It is a tremendous amount, it boggles the mind', said a knowing attorney involved with one of the plaintiffs in another matter (Cornwell 1996: 271). If any one payee spilled the beans all would lose their compensation—just as the judge handed the case to the jury for its verdict on Lilly's seemingly obvious culpability. Lilly paid privately, or was ordered to pay publicly, in several other drug cases: Oraflex (for arthritis) in 1982 after 28 deaths and a great many who suffered liver and kidney damage; and in 2009 paid out the largest ever liability sum, US$1.42 billion, following 8,000 lawsuits (involving 26,000 cases) for its handling of the schizophrenia drug Zyprexa (Corporate Research Project, Phillip Mattera, 27 August 2014, online). Such is the power of this corporation that Zyprexa is still on the market. And Lilly still advertises its good practices and ethical values in the face of more than a dozen court judgments against it for bribery, racial discrimination in employment, wilful environmental damage, fudging trials, false claims, withholding vital patient information, serious tax and subsidy dodges and anti-competitive practices. So, we should ask why does the medical profession continue to prescribe Zyprexa?

There is another aspect to this realm of medication: in our concluding chapter, we give some details of the extent which these therapeutic pharmaceuticals are the medium by which persons take their own lives.

The other side effect of a world suffering multiple disorders is that crime and punishment have taken a backward step, or leap, to be replaced by illness and therapy in our new *Erewhon*. In the middle of the nineteenth century, Britain's House of Lords

---

[5]In 2007, the FDA admitted that 'SSRIs can cause madness at all ages and that the drugs are very dangerous': see 'Antidepressants and murder: case not closed', *BMJ* (2017) 358 https://doi.org/10. 1136/bmj.j3697 (Published 02 August, cite this as: BMJ 2017; 358: j3697).

established the M'Naghten (or Macnaughten) Rules which, among other things, stated that 'to establish a defence on the ground of insanity it must be clearly proven that, at the time of committing the act, the accused was labouring under such a defect of reason, from disease of the mind, as not to know the nature and quality of the act he was doing or, if he did know it, that he did not know it was wrong (Walker 1980: 792–793). 'And so, Your Honour, my client Billy suffers seven of the DSM-5 disorders. The real Billy didn't do it—because he's basically a good sort but the stress got to him, he wasn't himself, he was beside himself, anxious, he smokes dope, he's tried methamphetamine, he's an abused child with gin-soaked parents and he hadn't taken his meds. We ask that he be given counselling therapy'.

The ever-increasing suicide prevention programs disappoint. They don't distinguish suicide from illness, as discussed in Chap. 6. While they differentiate between prevention strategies they don't differentiate between suicide *genre*s or *categories*. Suicide isn't measles, smallpox or polio and no vaccinations are to hand, and it isn't one virus or bacterium. In this context, *prevention* is a pretentious word, inferring that preventionists know all about the phenomenon, understand it, can deal with it, and can *forestall* it. We all need to think seriously about choosing to use words like alleviation, mitigation, deflection, deferment—to be more realistic, and to avoid failure as a result of unachievable aims. (Intervention is something different. Crisis supports, counselling and emergency interdictions for those who reach out is in another category.) Furthermore, statistics are unreliable and under-reporting remains idiosyncratic despite improved coronial practices. Unhelpfully, coroners may not presume suicide, even in the most obvious of cases, and the levels of proof required by coroners differ widely (see Chap. 10). And since the official rates slither up and down and sideways like quicksilver, talking about halving or reducing or eliminating suicide by prevention agencies is chasing after a *chimera*, that shape-shifting monster of Greek mythology.

In this book, we look briefly at the place of suicide in society from antiquity to the Middle Ages, at what philosophers had to say about it, and suicide as 'science' in the present day. It takes on board the vexing question of the impact of the suicide's action: the matter of rejection. Has society rejected the suicide or is our outrage and upset at the phenomenon because the suicide has rejected *us*?

What do we really know about the statistical base on which *all* suicide study rests—the collectivity of coronial determinations? Is it likely that Hungarians are 17 times more prone to suicide than Mexicans? Or is there a connection between the religions of those countries and their willingness to determine suicide? Eastern Orthodoxy remains vehement about the gross sinfulness of suicide, hence the low rate of suicide in Greece (or the unwillingness of coroners to find such verdicts?) Are the rates as alarming as we believe them to be, or are they really twice as bad? The latter, it seems. That question leads to another: why is it that suicide, especially among the young, is such a grim and gross social indicator even in the face of the youth who die by drug abuse, excessive alcohol and reckless actions?

We all know about cancer, and fear it. We also know that that disease has many forms, and we have professionals who specialise in addressing those quite divergent categories. So why do we insist and persist in treating suicide as monolithic? Why aren't we better able to differentiate the age cohorts, the genres, the types of suicide and the groups most at risk? Why do our prevention agencies address the 8-year-old Aboriginal girl in the remote Kimberley region of Western Australia in the same or similar way as the drought-stricken, near-bankrupt, recently widowed 70-year-old farmer in parched western New South Wales? Do agencies ever consider Durkheim's work on social cohesion? Or Baechler's quartet that seeks to pinpoint motives like aggression or escapism or gambling with one's life? Given this enmeshment of suicide in the biomedical vision of the (Western) world, can we bring ourselves to conceive of something called 'rational suicide'? We doubt it: for now, it goes against the whole grain and holy writ of suicide as 'depression, depression, depression' (Goldney 2003).

Is Aboriginal suicide different from mainstream suicide? Certainly it is, despite the howls of protest from those who are intent on locating a suicide gene, or chemical imbalances in the brain, and who abjure all considerations of history, geography, anthropology, sociology and ecology (admittedly, topics in which they probably have not been educated). Is mainstream society suicide different from the Aboriginal case? Yes, at least in the senses of age cohorts, at-risk factors, historical background and, something almost totally ignored, *political* contexts.

We have a goodly number of prevention organisations and strategies in Australia. But what do we know about them? Which agencies are undertaking or are entrusted with addressing suicide? Who runs them? Are they formally trained? Who funds them? Is the constant clamour for more money *the* answer to what is deemed an urgent problem? Is the evidence that more SANE ambassadors, more beyondblue 'awareness' advertising, more anti-stigma campaigns are reducing suicide attempts and completions? How are these organisations and programs evaluated and made accountable? What is the evidence that these suicide prevention strategies have eased, halved or even ameliorated suicide? And why are they so opposed to questioning, let alone challenging, the vested interests and existing programs and funded policies on, among other public issues, suicide?

Has education—always seen as the magic panacea that cures all things—altered the state of affairs that we perceive as so unacceptable, so confronting? No: the rates escalate, for all manner of reasons, as will be discussed. Have the large sums expended on suicide prevention had any positive outcomes? Do we need another despairing cliché that 'further research is needed' in the biomedical field? (Certainly more is needed into the social contexts of suicide.)

Is there any validity in the assertion that 'good works' should never be questioned—because of their inherent good intent? Professor Ian Hickie, psychiatrist, advocate and a commissioner on Australia's National Mental Health Commission, viewed the current situation fragmented, dysfunctional and unmonitored, 'throwing good money after bad'. But he lamented that some of these agencies 'are divorced from clinical services as if suicidal people don't have mental health problems' (Hickie 2017).

Our coronial systems have undergone some major changes in the first decades of this century. But has coronial determination on the matter of suicide really improved with the appointment of magistrates (only) as coroners? These questions are addressed in later chapters.

References

Alvarez, A. (1974). *The Savage God*. London: Penguin Books.

Baechler, J. (1975). *Suicides*. New York: Basic Books.

Bentall, R. (2009). *Doctoring the mind: Why psychiatric treatments fail*. London: Penguin Books.

Burton, N. (2015). https://www.psychologytoday.com/us/blog/hide-and-seek/201509/when-homosexuality-stopped-being-mental-disorder.

Butler, S. (1872). *Erewhon*. London: Trübner and Ballantyne.

Cornwell, J. (1996). *The power to harm: Mind, medicine, and murder on trial*. London: Viking.

Corporate Research Project, Phillip Mattera, August 27, 2014. (Online).

Foucault, M. (2003). *Power: The essential Foucault: Selections from the essential works of Foucault, 1954–1984*. London: Penguin Books.

Frankl, V. (Ed.). ([1946], 1984) *Man's search for meaning*. New York: Washington Square Press.

Goldney, R. (2003). Depression and suicidal behavior: The real estate analogy. *Crisis: The Journal of Crisis Intervention and Suicide Prevention, 24*(2), 87–88.

Gregory, R. L. (Ed.). (1987). *The Oxford companion to the mind*. New York: Oxford University Press.

Hickie, I. (2017). Putting mental health services and suicide prevention reform into practice. *Public Health Research Practice, 27*(2), e2721710. http://dx.doi.org/10.17061/phrp2721710.

Hobsbawm, E. (1998). *Uncommon people: Resistance, rebellion and jazz*. New York: The New Press.

Horwitz, A. & Wakefield, J. (2007). *The loss of sadness: How psychiatry transformed normal sorrow into depressive disorder*. New York: Oxford University Press.

Kreitman, N. (1987). Parasuicide in Gregory, Richard L. (ed). *The Oxford companion to the mind*. Oxford: Oxford University Press.

Lieberman, J. (2015). *Shrinks: The untold story of psychiatry*. New York: Little, Brown Company.

Marsh, I. (2010). *Suicide: Foucault, history and truth*. Cambridge, UK: Cambridge University Press.

Robertson, M., Light, E., Lipworth, W., & Walter, G. (2017). Psychiatry, genocide and the National Socialist state: Lessons learnt, ignored and forgotten. In N. Marczak & K. Shields (Eds.), *Genocide perspectives V*. Sydney: UTSePress.

Rodwell, G. (1998). 'If the feeble-minded are to be preserved ...', Special education and eugenics in Tasmania 1900–1930. *Issues in Educational Research, 8*(2), 131–156.

Solnit, R. (2009). *'A paradise built in hell', the extraordinary communities that arise in disasters*. New York: Penguin Books.

Szasz, T. (1974). *The secret sin*. New York: Anchor Books.

Szasz, T. (1997). *The manufacture of madness: A comparative study of the inquisition and the mental health movement*. Syracuse, NY: Syracuse University Press.

Szasz, T. (1998). *Fatal freedom: The ethics and politics of suicide*. Santa Barbara, CA: Praeger Publishers.

Szasz, T. (2007). *The medicalization of everyday life: Selected essays*. Syracuse, NY: Syracuse University Press.

Tatz, C. (2017). *Australia's unthinkable genocide*. Bloomington, IN: Xlibris.

Walker, D. M. (1980). *The Oxford companion to law*. Oxford: Clarendon Press.
Wekstein, L. (1979). *Handbook of suicidology: Principles, problems, and practice*. New York: Bruner/Mazel Publishers.
White, J., Marsh, I., Kral, M., & Morris, J. (Eds.). (2016). *Critical suicidology: Transforming suicide research and prevention for the 21st century*. Vancouver: UBC Press.
Winkler v Eli Lilly; Potter v Eli Lilly.
Wylie, P. (1942). *Generation of vipers*. London: Frederick Muller Limited.

Chapter 4
History Lessons

*An historical approach makes it possible to see suicide in
different temporal contexts and to try to understand the meaning
it has for people of varying backgrounds and experiences.*

—George Rosen (1975) [George Rosen (1910–1977) was
professor of the history of medicine at Yale University]

*I believe that no man ever threw away life while it was worth
keeping.*

—David Hume (1757) [Scottish philosopher and historian,
considered the father of social science (1711–1776)]

Abstract The universality of suicide in human affairs; suicide in the Bible and in the
Graeco–Roman world; tolerance replaced by Christian condemnation of suicide as
a cardinal sin; criminalisation of suicide and forfeiture of a suicider's assets to government treasuries; bizarre burial practices; the Renaissance and significant French
studies of suicide.

Keywords Suicide texts · From badness to madness

'Ours', we assert, 'is a new world'. That was then and this is now, a condemnatory
point made by the late political scientist Tony Judt. It is a nice phrasing of the reality
that we live in an historical era, perhaps an anti-historical one, where memory is last
year and all that matters is now. *Then*, the past, comes across as quaint, a collection
of curiosities. The British novelist L. P. Hartley (1895–1972) is frequently quoted:
'the past is a foreign country, they do things differently there' (Hartley 1953). Our
country doesn't like that country and we don't care for the lessons of the past,
especially the ignominious or uncomfortable yesteryears. The present, of course,
rarely exists without a past and if ever a subject was in need of historical context, it is
suicide. The shame and stigma of the very word, the brutal laws and bizarre burials
didn't arrive from outer space, let alone leave on the starship.

© Springer Nature Switzerland AG 2019   31
C. Tatz and S. Tatz, *The Sealed Box of Suicide*,
https://doi.org/10.1007/978-3-030-28159-5_4

History, among other things, is a chronology of significant events, an aggregate of things that happened. Whatever else suicide may be, it is an eternal behaviour and it can only be understood through looking, however briefly, at the ages and phases of the practice. Society can only address the many facets that make up suicide if there is some understanding of why, and what, it is. Merely explicating, comparing, and analysing suicide doesn't provide perception or comprehension. Much of today's discourse on self-death conveys, wittingly or not, a feeling of an epidemic invasion, an external, recent and sudden 'attack' on a society dedicated to the pursuit of happiness and long life, an affliction that arises in the unwell, in the 'crooked' who are in need of 'straightening' [as English novelist Samuel Butler informed us in 1872]. During the Australian federal election campaign of 2019, the conservative prime minister insisted that youth suicide is 'a curse'—evoking a mediaeval notion of Satanic evil—and later vowed his government would be 'curse-breakers' of suicide (which entails an expansion of psychiatric and psychological services).[1] More often than not, suicide has a sociopolitical context. The suicide canvas, however large, needs exploring to its very edges, to its essential paint admixtures. That must include forays into suicide practices that arise from degrees of conformity in any society, obedience, acquiescence, submission, compliance, veneration of traditional culture and fear. Those triggers are normal emotions, not signs or signals of mental illness, let alone an invasive virus.

Medicine is replete with fads and foibles that were the order of the day one day and gone the next—eager to make way for 'the latest' in technology and therapy, with neither a blink nor a blush at the crassness or wrongness of what has only just been superseded. The British First Fleet took possession of Australia in 1788 in the name of King George III, at the very height of His Majesty undergoing leeches, cupping, blistering, purgatives and emetics at least three times daily. He probably suffered from porphyria [an illness of the nervous system] but medicine of the day insisted it was 'all in the stools'—which were collected, weighed, assayed, prodded, sniffed and pronounced upon by the hour. In our time, we have witnessed ingestion of apricot kernels at one end and coffee enemas at the other as the way to treat cancer (Rosenbaum 2001).

When looking for references to suicide, particularly through Internet search engines, the usual opening is a discussion of mental illness of one kind or another: depression, bipolar disorder, personality disorder, schizophrenia and post-traumatic stress. Next comes a set of at-risk factors—financial difficulties, broken relationships, sexual identity, bullying, alcoholism, sedative addictions, a family history of self-harm and depletion of brain hormones. On occasion, existential themes arising from religion and philosophy are 'associated', whereas those themes should be at the very bases of the suicide phenomenon. In an essentially Eurocentric literature, little attention is given to the eras where suicide was praiseworthy in some societies and

---

[1] *The Guardian* (Australia), 13 April 2019.

obligatory in others (as in Hindu, Chinese and Japanese cultures). In some ancient world cultures suicide was even considered a patriotic act. That was both then and now.

Western thinkers once believed that 'primitive' people didn't suicide because they had nothing complex and convoluted to be disturbed about. Anthropologists— among others Franz Boas and Bronislaw Malinowski—have indeed shown high rates of suicide among native peoples as a response to shame, dishonour, to avoid curses coming to fruition, as revenge, to avoid ageing, to allow younger people access to scarce food resources, and so on. Many tribal people admired suicide as a solution; others deplored the practice; some, including Australian Aborigines, were said to have found the very idea 'laughable' (Sir George Grey[2] in Dublin and Bunzel 1933: 138). Rarely do we read of the historic mass suicides of despair, like the Colombian and other South American tribes who jumped from cliffs rather than face Spanish colonisation. David Stannard's *American Holocaust* (1993) is a near-unreadable account of the genocidal atrocities and the native peoples' responses. [We discuss the suicide of ethnic despair in Chap. 6.] Interest in the causes of suicide has long overtaken concerns about the ethics of suicide, leaving self-death as if a modern phenomenon, a medical one, an epidemic of recency that needs combating.

4.1 Some Texts

The history of suicide reflects the history of mankind, wrote Louis Wekstein (1997: 22), and we are fortunate to have some seminal texts on that interconnection. For traditional history purposes, one can start with the very readable work of poet, novelist and critic Al Alvarez, *The Savage God: A Study of Suicide* (1974). Written as a form of eulogy to his late friend and suicider, the poet Sylvia Plath, it is a masterly account of some of the theories and practices of Western suicide. For him (and for us), suicide is like a dye that permeates Western society and cannot be washed out. Other good sources are Seymour Perlin's *A Handbook for the Study of Suicide* (1975), Marzio Barbagli's *Farewell to the World: A History of Suicide* (2015) and Jennifer Michael Hecht's *Stay: A History of Suicide and Philosophies Against It* (2013). Her chapter on the two great voices on suicide in the twentieth century—Émile Durkheim and Albert Camus—is essential reading. Perlin's *Handbook* does what any comprehensive book should do: it examines suicide from the perspectives of history, philosophy, literature, anthropology, sociology, biology and epidemiology. A recurring theme of our book is that to be understood, suicide needs every ounce of holism and interdisciplinary lenses it can find, not more micrograms of particularism.

But if one is to comprehend the legacies of shame, stigma and taboo that suffuses suicide in society and that lingers in the legal system, then Alexander Murray's two

---

[2]Governor of South Australia, 1841–1845.

volumes—*Suicide in the Middle Ages*—are the significant books. Volume I is 'The Violent Against Themselves' (1998) and Volume II is tellingly named 'The Curse on Self-Murder' (2000). Murray's work is history at its best: illuminating, invigorating and taking us through the chronicles that lie beneath most of today's attitudes on concealment, shame, stigma and euphemism. Georges Minois' *History of Suicide* (2001) gives us insight into cultural factors and influences of suicide in England and France. Margaret Pabst Battin's *The Ethics of Suicide* (2015) is a monumental documentary source book which one can dip into and browse across the centuries (2015). These works provide the essential contexts of suicide—political, religious and social systems, not merely the attempted post-mortem reconstruction of how or even why the deceased is on the pathologist's mortuary table.

We can always refer to Sigmund Freud (1856–1939) and his view—in his *The Psychopathology of Everyday Living* (1901)—about the 'subconscious drive for suicide'. Benjamin Franklin (1706–1790) touched on this a hundred years earlier, with his assertion that 'nine men in ten are would-be suicides'.

The French sociologist Jean Baechler said that 'the literature on suicide has something of the monstrous about it' when one looks at the extent of the titles on the subject (Baechler 1979: 3).[3] Suicide, he wrote, 'is the most unremittingly studied human behaviour'. Just as one needs to read Durkheim, so Baechler on *Suicides* is essential. To which we add Jack Douglas' *The Social Meanings of Suicide* (1967).

In sum, we argue that the best sources of education about self-death are to be found in the philosophers and earlier social scientists rather than medical-centred materials. Alvarez's book focuses on the late Sylvia Plath and her genre of confessional poetry. He was much taken by the suicide themes of poets like Dante, Cowper, Donne and Chatterton. One looks in vain for a better class of more modern writing on the subject. Much of the material comes across as simplistic doggerel as in this snippet from American songwriter and thriller novelist Dan Brown[4]:

> It isn't brave, and it isn't clever,
> To inflict pain on other people forever.
> Life isn't all about you.
> Your life isn't all about you.
> That rope hangs your family too,
> and those pills kill your friends.
> The pain, hurt and upset
> doesn't stop when your life ends.
> So please don't do it.

---

[3]In 1927, the German researcher Hans Rost published a suicide bibliography of 3,750 titles. See also the David Lester and Sell guide to suicide information (1980).

[4]'A Note on Suicide' in PoemHunter.com.

4.2 Greece and Rome

The Graeco–Roman world, the one sometimes called 'classical civilisation', had much to offer: their ideas on culture, law, architecture, road works, water systems, engineering, public health, mental health and social systems. Roman law—always imbued with the dictates of natural law and right reason—neither forbade nor condemned suicide. There was serious discussion on the role and place of self-death. There was admiration for some of the great men of the day who took their lives— Hannibal (probably by poison in 183 BCE), Socrates, Cato the Younger, Seneca the Younger, and Caesar's assassin, Brutus. Aristotle and Pythagoras didn't approve for pragmatic reasons, seeing suicide as reducing the quantum of valued members of society.

Greeks and Romans condoned suicide as an honourable and legitimate way out of humiliation, capture, and certain death on a battlefield. Common enough was the practice of a body of soldiers to take their lives when their military leader died, was killed or suicided. Loyalty suicide of this kind came close to being a ritual. Herodotus described the Thracians as having a ritual in which the woman adjudged the most loved (in that polygamous society) was chosen to die on the funeral pyre of the dead husband (Perlin 1975: 6). Suicide was also viewed as a sensible form of euthanasia. Martyrdom or seeking martyrdom was often expressed by self-destruction, especially among Christians; suicide was seen as a 'prize' snatched from the wickedness of evil men. More or less contemporaneous with early Christianity, other faiths—like Stoicism and Epicureanism—saw sense in suicide even while they didn't champion it. Zeno, the founder of Stoicism, stated that 'the wise man for reasonable cause will make his own exit'—to honour his country, for the sake of his friends or because he suffers intolerable pain (Perlin 1975: 10).

Stoicism, founded in Greek philosophy and adopted by the Romans, is a concept that inspires myriad interpretations. Above all, it emphasises rationalism and logic. Stoics viewed the world as unpredictable, with human beings unable to control external factors. For them, humans must make the right ethical choices about their behaviour—it is not what happens to individuals but how they react to these events. This is a logical approach to the world founded in rational decision-making, where reason champions emotion, and happiness is gained not through the accumulation of wealth, objects or even love but by understanding the universe and where individuals are placed within it. Stoic philosophy equated an individual's alignment of nature with happiness. Stoics viewed suicide with a degree of tolerance.

In that era, suicide belonged within the realms of heroism and self-sacrifice. Suicide was certainly a feature in ancient and classical times. Dublin and Bunzel established that suicide was popular in ancient Rome and surrounding countries: 'In ancient times certain warlike peoples, such as the Germans, Scandinavians, and ancient Gauls, regarded suicide as highly courageous and noble' (Dublin and Bunzel 1933: 145).

The great Roman statesman and philosopher Cicero (106–43 BCE) was much taken with Stoicism and through them he brought a new understanding of suicide, and mental illness, to Rome. Cicero praised the suicide of Cato, who stabbed himself to death rather than live under the despotic rule of Caesar. Cicero examined mental disorders in *The Tusculan Disputations* (Nordenfelt 1997). He approved of the unique Stoic view: that while life must be suffered, and reason and virtue guide the individual, suicide delivered an acceptable end to pain and dotage, an end without stigma or shame once all reasoning and considerations had been evaluated. In *De Finibus*, Cicero said: 'When a man's circumstances contain a preponderance of things in accordance with nature, it is appropriate for him to remain alive; when he possesses or sees in prospect a majority of the contrary things, it is appropriate for him to depart from life. This makes it plain that it is on occasion appropriate for the Wise Man to quit life although he is happy, and also of the Foolish Man to remain in life although he is miserable' (Loeb Classic Library 1931: 281). Pliny the Elder (Gaius Plinius Secundus, 23–79 CE) and Gaius Pliny the Younger (Plinius Caecilius Secundus, 61–113 CE) wrote what is interpreted as favourably or understandably about suicide.

Some weird practices operated even though no penalties were established. Though suicide was tolerated generally, in Athens a suicider's hand was chopped off, especially the one that did the deed, and an honourable burial was denied. In Italy, suicide was only penalised if committed by criminals, soldiers and slaves. 'Mental illness' of a kind was recognised—for example, menstrual pain symptoms were regarded as such illness. Physicians of the day recognised that violent people were wont to injure themselves and prescribed restraints for those so afflicted.

Self-killing was very much associated with honour, especially after the rape (and subsequent suicide) of the chaste Lucretia in 510 BCE, an event that led to the overthrow of the Roman monarchy. Her suicide inspired art by Titian, Botticelli, Rembrandt, Dürer and literary works by Dante, Chaucer and Shakespeare.

Hecht, among other scholars, talked about both mythical and historical suicide in the Graeco–Roman world. In both forms, she wrote, the categories were pretty clear: altruistic suicide, suicide because of great loss, suicide because of shame and suicide because of love gone wrong (Hecht 2013: 18). Among many others, Shakespearean audiences in the sixteenth century (and in the centuries since then) understood why Romeo, Juliet, Lady Macbeth, Othello, Ophelia and Mark Anthony took their lives and why the Prince of Denmark aired the possibility.

In those ancient days, there was evidence of people, often young people, resentful of the world. Seneca the Elder (5 BCE–65 CE) called this *displicentia sui*, self-dissatisfaction and recognised that this feeling took the form of self-harm and even suicide.

In Chap. 1, we mentioned the handful of Old Testament suicides, not one of which attracts biblical commentary or condemnation. The historian Josephus did comment on the mass suicide at Masada, saying that 'for those who have laid mad hands upon themselves', 'the darkest regions of the nether world will receive their souls' (Perlin 1975: 5). But Josephus did concede that suicide in defence of the Torah was justifiable in all circumstances. It is interesting that this historian used the word 'mad' in a politico-religious context.

Christianity began as a tolerated faith; later, it became the state faith. At first, the Christian opposition to suicide was purely economical: if a slave suicided, one lost an asset. Second, a number of competing religions tolerated, even promoted, suicide, and Christianity sought to differentiate itself. In 563 CE, suicide was formally condemned but it took until 1284 for suicide burials in consecrated grounds to be forbidden.

Christianity came to deplore what it called the ancient world's pagan superstitions, yet that new religion was replete with 'knowledge' based on ignorance, magic, miracles, irrationality and a dark imagination. It wasn't simply that the Devil was omnipresent. It was a 'fact' that people who took their lives had made pacts with Satan, the very creature who was embodied in Jews, a people depicted (at least from the thirteenth century) with horns, tails, and cloven hooves, people who fornicated with pigs and brought plagues to the people and blight to their crops.

Earlier, we discussed St Augustine's sinfulness of suicide. Here, it is worth adding the comments of another great Catholic thinker, St Thomas Aquinas (1225–1274). He had seemingly secular reasons against suicide. First, 'killing oneself is contrary to natural inclination'. Second, parts belong to a whole, and any suicide is a detraction from the community and an injustice to that community. Third, and familiarly in the Judeo-Christian traditions, only God kills and makes one live: He has sole jurisdiction (in Battin 2015: 229).

St Augustine and then Aquinas epitomised Catholic canon on suicide as the ultimate sin, but Sir Thomas Moore (1478–1535) was to be the voice of reason on the subject. In his *Utopia*, published in 1516, he wrote much in the manner of many moderns, including Jean Améry, (Battin 2015: 239):

> The sick (as I said) they see to with great affection, and let nothing at all pass concerning either physic or good diet, whereby they may be restored again to their health. Such as be sick of incurable disease they comfort with sitting with them, with talking with them, and, to be short, with all manner of help that be. But if the disease be not only incurable, but also full of continual pain and anguish, then the priests and the magistrates exhort the man (since he is not able to do any duty in life and by overliving his own death and is noisome and irksome and grievous to himself), that he will determine with himself no longer to cherish that pestilential and painful disease. And, seeing his life is to him but a torment, that he will not be unwilling to die but rather take a good hope to him, but dispatch himself out of that painful life as out of a prison or a rack of torture, or else suffer himself willingly to be rid of it by other. And in so doing they tell him he shall do wisely seeing by his death he shall lose no commodity, but end his pain.

The change in epochs between the ancient and the mediaeval worlds, the light and the dark ages, was remarkable—and for the worse. Here, we don't address the many aspects of suicide across the millennia, but rather touch briefly on the transition from some enlightenment and rationality on the subject to its decree as the ultimate sin, then to its declaration as criminal, its punishment, its affirmation as insanity, then to the more euphemistic 'mental illness', and to today's 'tragic event' and 'epidemic'. (We need a reminder that a mere 60 years ago in England a man named Lionel Henry Churchill was imprisoned for six months for trying to put a bullet in his head after being found alongside his decomposing wife. That was the era of the Richard Nixon–John F. Kennedy television debates, the big-time year of Elvis Presley and Cliff Richard in the pop world, the Rome Olympics, the capture of the Nazi Adolf Eichmann.)[5] Sociologists have delved into the external factors, the social forces that affect the suicide act; psychologists and psychiatrists have concentrated on intrapsychic conflicts of many kinds. Betwixt, so to speak, there have been several historians, and it is in that history that we may well find a greater insight into Camus' 'only philosophical problem'.

4.3 Burials

For much of the Middle Ages (500–1500 CE) and even into the Renaissance era, suicide—always called self-murder rather than the later word *suicide*—was considered one of the lowest possible criminal acts in Britain: the suicide 'is drawn by a horse to the place of the punishment and shame, where he is hanged on a gibbet, and none may take the body down but by the authority of the magistrate' (Szasz 1974: 64). Burial was usually at night, at the crossroads, so that carriages would trample the dead, by now seen as a vampire; and if that were not enough, a stake was driven through the heart and a stone placed over the deceased's face—to prevent any rising. Suicides had 'non-burials', that is, they were interred without benefit of ceremonies and outside the location of consecrated ground: they were regarded as profane burials, taken *to the fields*, placed *under the gallows*, thrown into the *carrion pit*, placed *at the junction roads* or buried *under stones*. Commonly, the suicide's body was staked and decapitated (Murray, II 2000: 41–53). Louis XIV added another practice in 1670: the deceased was dragged through the streets, face down, then hung or laid out on the garbage dump. In England and some parts of Europe, a suicide was declared a *felo de se* ('a felon on himself'), his properties forfeited to the Crown rather than passing to his inheritors. This practice was abolished as late as 1882.

An older Code of Jewish Law also buried the suicide in 'the hock', an unconsecrated place and didn't offer prayers, tributes or eulogies to those who took their lives. Modern Jewish and Christian practice allow a suicide a 'regular' burial, taking a 'softer' approach if there are indications of mental illness, which in today's medical paradigm, there always are. Progressive Judaism now recognises cases where

---

[5] *BBC News* (20 August 2011) carried a report on the illegality of attempted suicide: a *Times* editorial of 1958 reported that there were 5,387 attempted suicides that year, of whom 613 were prosecuted and 33 sent to prison.

persons 'resort' to suicide because of unendurable pain, pain that distorts the rational mind—in which case the deceased has a normal burial.

4.4 Melancholia

Georges Minois' *History of Suicide* has an excellent depiction of how the French and English philosophers, early social scientists and churchmen viewed suicide. In short, badly. Their language of opposition was ferocious, to put it mildly. They inveighed, fulminated, ranted at the very idea of self-death, but they did spend much time on the topic. He quoted the French political philosopher Montesquieu (2015: 293):

> European laws are ferocious against those who kill themselves. They are, so to speak, made to die twice, for they are hauled ignominiously through the streets, proclaimed infamous, and their property is confiscated. It seems to me … that these laws are unjust. If I am laden with sorrow, misery, and contempt, why should anyone want to prevent me from putting an end to my cares and cruelly deprive me of a remedy which lies in my hands?

Good question from Montequieu in 1721 and as good a question today.

Melancholia, deriving from the Greek word for blackness of the bile, is also an old-fashioned word for clinical depression. A Franciscan monk of the thirteenth century, David of Augsburg, talked about three types of *acedia*, which he described (quoted in Perlin 1975: 12–13) as:

> The first is a certain bitterness of the mind which cannot be pleased by anything cheerful or wholesome. It feeds upon disgust and loathes human intercourse. This is what the Apostle calls the sorrow of the world that worketh death. It inclines to despair, diffidence, and suspicions, and sometimes drives its victim to suicide where he is oppressed by unreasonable grief. Such sorrow arises sometimes from previous impatience, sometimes from the fact that one's desire for some object has been delayed or frustrated and sometimes from the abundance of melancholic humours, in which case it behoves the physician rather than the priest to prescribe a remedy.

A brilliant quote, it is one that may well pinpoint the beginnings of the biomedical sovereignty over suicide. The Middle Ages presented two sources of suicidal inclination. One was a vice, prompted or promoted by the devil; the other was an emotional or mental state induced by an excess of the humours, like black bile. Up to the thirteenth century, ideas on suicide came from folklore and peasant beliefs, from ecclesiastical canons and medical opinions. In the middle of the fourteenth century, the legal authorities stepped in and suicide became a criminal matter.

4.5   Property

Many European states adopted the practice of confiscation, often called forfeiture, of a right, a privilege, property, and assets owned by a person who committed treason, suppressed knowledge of intended treason, murder or suicide. An 'ordinary' suicider forfeited his goods, while a suicider who took their life to avoid a felony conviction lost both their goods and their land. Four centuries later, in 1870 in England, the *Forfeiture Act* abolished confiscation in cases of murder, treason and suicide. Thus ended a long period in which suicide was dealt with by forfeiture of assets, burial anywhere but in consecrated ground, degradation of the corpses and criminal punishment if one survived the attempt.

Before that law was changed, lawyers invented a legal fiction as a protection against a ludicrous statute which not only deprived a suicider of the right to bequeath but also denied them a religious burial. It formulated the idea that a suicider was 'of unsound mind' and didn't know what they were doing, but that a guardian or curator of 'sound mind' was perfectly able to administer the assets and estates of the dead one. We need to remember that the lawyers, not the doctors, devised the solution, the fiction that suicide occurred because 'the balance of his mind was disturbed'.

What was once a mortal sin and a criminal offence became a private vice, something shameful, kept in the closet, something, if at all possible, not mentioned; as Alvarez put it, 'less self-slaughter than self-abuse'. Murray has written much on the era of euphemism: he didn't kill himself but rather, 'he raised his hand against himself'. Stigma always attached. Szasz made a good point when he argued that the holy grail of scientists, 'objective' research and 'objective' language, betrays strong emotions: abortion is called murder or foeticide by those who disapprove of it; it is called birth control by those who approve. Why not 'death control', he asked, by those who seek it rather than the negative term 'suicide'.

4.6   The Renaissance

From the sixteenth to the eighteenth centuries, this ubiquitous behaviour was named and defined in differing ways. Nearly all dictionaries come back to the Latin, the killing of self. Germans used *selbstvernichtung*, self-destruction and *selbstmord*, the latter term immediately implying that a crime (of murder) had been committed. Of interest is that the word *suicide* first appeared in English in the seventeenth century, used by Sir Thomas Browne in 1637 (Murray, I 1998: 38).

Attitudes began to change at this time, at least in the English Renaissance period in the sixteenth century. But it was, rather, the influential father of the essay form, the Frenchman Michel de Montaigne (1533–1592), who brought humanism and scepticism to the reading public. He was not pro-suicide in general but wrote about 'unendurable pain' and 'fear of a worse death' as justification for the act (Battin 2015: 278–279). Christian humanism, enlightened philosophy, and some powerful theological minds led to a less condemnatory approach. John Donne's *Biathanatos*, published in 1644 (36 years after he wrote it), defended suicide. The act, he declared, was not incompatible with the laws of God, reason and nature. Robert Burton's encyclopaedic *Anatomy of Melancholy* (1621) recognised the relationship between melancholy and suicide and 'after many tedious days', at last, the sufferers, by drowning, hanging 'or some such fearful end, make away with themselves' (Perlin 1975: 17).

Two clergymen, the German Johannes Neser (in 1613) and the Englishman John Sym (in 1637), published what they saw as preventive texts. Both differentiated between those who could enjoy salvation and those suiciders who couldn't: the former, afflicted with melancholy, inner conflicts, gout and stones in the bladder, were saveable; the others were damned. Such distinctions, however simplistic, at least showed a movement towards understanding the phenomenon.

Montesquieu (1689–1755), the eminent Frenchman of the Enlightenment, wrote at length about the 'principled' and comprehensible suicide of the Romans and the 'unaccountable' self-demise of the English. Like other writers of his time, he believed that environment was a contributing factor. The English lived in a gloomy, melancholic-making environ, the Romans (obviously) in a sunnier place. (A glance at our Appendix shows that the top 11 suicide nations are cold places and the last eight on the world table are hot ones. A possible link but one that needs caution and careful study.)

The great men of the Enlightenment—Hume, Beccaria, Rousseau, Voltaire—were strongly opposed to the traditional Christian attitude to suicide, asserting a secular attitude to the matter. An English physician, George Cheyne, published *The English Malady* in 1733. His focus on the individual contributed to the work of William Battie, whose *A Treatise on Madness* was published in 1758:

> Whatever may be the cause of Anxiety, it chiefly discovers itself by that agonising impatience observable in some men of black November days, of easterly winds, of heat, cold, damps etc. Which real misery of theirs is sometimes derided by dull mortals as a whimsical affectation. And of the same nature are the perpetual tempests of love, hatred, and other turbulents provoked by nothing or at most by very trifles. In which state of habitual diseases many drag on their wretched lives; whilst others, unequal to evils of which they see no remedy but death, rarely resolve to end them at any rate. Which very frequent cases of suicide though generally ascribed to lunacy by the verdict of a good-natured jury, except where the deceased hath not left assets, are no more entitled to the benefit of passing for pardonable acts of madness than he who deliberately has killed the man he hated deserves be acquitted as not knowing what he did (in Perlin 1975: 21).

These works are significant because they signal, in their way, that critical thinkers were now beginning to look at suicide as some form of madness rather than baseness and badness. In the eighteenth century, hypochondria was an 'issue', the talk of the day and several men began to make connections between that condition and suicide. Richard Blackmoore defined hypochondria as resulting from a 'morbid constitution of the spirits' and Richard Whytt concluded 'depression, despair, melancholia, or even madness' among the symptoms of hypochondria. In 1775, Michael Alberti established a link between hypochondria and a desire for death (Minois: 243). The world was on its way to the medicalisation of suicide.

In the nineteenth century, investigations on suicide took two forms, both relevant today. One was the statistical-sociological approach, the other the medico-psychiatric perspective. The most impressive work of the era was formulated in France in correlating diseases of the body with disease of the mind, with investigations of the relationship of suicide to climate, gender, age, broken relationships, family, heredity, insanity, the brain. All this culminated in Durkheim looking at the nature of society and the regulation of nation states.

Before Durkheim came a renowned French physician, Jean-Etiene Esquirol (1772–1840), a humanist who reformed the administration of asylums, sought personal interaction of patients and doctors and had patients eat at his family table. He was among the first to establish systematic empirical observations of the mentally ill and define the difference between mental retardation and insanity. He distinguished between biological and behavioural disorders, between emotional disturbances and organic brain damage (Battin 2015: 475–476). The importance of Esquirol is that while he saw suicide as a result of insanity, he did not perceive suicide as a disease (Perlin 1975: 24). He wrote:

> Self-murder takes place under circumstances so opposite, and is determined by motives so diverse, that it cannot be limited to any single determination. However varied be the motives and the circumstances, which cause men to expose their lives, and to brave death, they almost always exalt the imagination, either on account of a good, more precious than life or an evil more formidable than death … Suicide is only a phenomenon, consecutive to a great number of diverse causes; that it presents itself under very different characters; and that this phenomenon is not exclusively confined to any one malady … It is in consequence of having made suicide a malady *sui generis* that they have developed general propositions, which experience disproves …

By the nineteenth century, at least in Britain, suicide was becoming less of a moral and religious question and more of a social and medical matter. The label of insanity became preferable to the disgrace attaching to someone who wittingly ended their life. By the time we get to the twenty-first century, mental illness is not only the norm but one that almost instantly produces sympathy, often empathy, and vigorous nods of 'understanding'.

Suicide ceased being criminal in Britain in 1961, in Australian states between 23 and 62 years ago,[6] and in Ireland in 1993. By the 1980s, 30 states in the USA had

---

[6]Tasmania in 1957, Victoria in 1967, Western Australia in 1972, Queensland in 1979, South Australia in 1983, Australian Capital Territory in 1990, New South Wales in 1993, and the Northern Territory in 1996.

no criminal statutes on suicide, though suicide is held to be a common law crime in some American jurisdictions. Suicide as disturbed balance of the mind was to become, and remain, the domain of the psychiatrists, the clinical psychologists, a few sociologists and social workers, and a great many statisticians. With 'depression' and 'stress' now bywords in our Western society, suicide is seen as the extreme of both, and hence even more the domain of those who deal in these matters and who are in a position to prescribe antidepressants or even more drastic 'therapies'.

There are several logical slippages in these perspectives of psychiatric and pharmaceutical treatment of 'depression'. For example, it is commonly claimed that at least up to a third of the population suffers from some form of anxiety, stress and depression in their lifetime[7]; that depression is a primary cause of suicide; and, therefore, this huge proportion of the population is at risk of committing suicide. This is patently untrue. Or, again, it is claimed that depression is *a*, if not *the*, major mental health risk factor in suicide; that antidepressants alleviate or control depression; and that the suicide rate therefore falls markedly across Australia when depression is treated. This again is a nonsensical claim.

Medication may stifle or deflect a suicide in many, and it may cause or enable suicide in others, but this does not mean that the 'depression' is, of itself, the cause of the suicidal impulse. There remains, however, a strong lay (and, regrettably, a medical) perception that the right pill will always solve the problem.

The nineteenth century label of 'unsound mind' left the burden of suicide, in all its manifestations and consequences, with the health professions. No one else wanted it and, surprisingly, the church was relieved to be absolved of an insoluble 'moral' and 'mortal' problem.

Suicide, as this brief chronicle shows, has gone through any number of phases, treatments, punishments, legal controls, philosophic permutations, moral judgments, religious reforms and geographical shifts. While social systems have changed and while science has developed in once unimaginable ways, one phenomenon has not changed: people kill themselves, make their own exit for their own reasons. Like Camus, we see this as a philosophical problem, beyond the reach of medicine.

References

Alvarez, A. (1974). *The Savage God: A study of suicide*. London: Penguin Books.
Baechler, J. (1979). *Suicides*. New York: Basic Books.
Barbagli, M. (2015). *Farewell to the world: A history of suicide*. New Jersey: Wiley.
Battin, M. P. (2015). *The ethics of suicide: Historical sources*. Oxford: Oxford University Press.
Burton, R. ([1621/1628] (1994)). *Anatomy of melancholy* (3 Vols.). Oxford: Oxford University Press.

---

[7] See https://www.beyondblue.org.au/media/statistics.

Cheyne, G. (1733). *The English malady: Or, a treatise of nervous diseases of all kinds, as spleen, vapours, lowness of spirits, hypochondriacal, and hysterical distempers, etc.* London: Strahan.

Douglas, J. (1967). *The social meanings of suicide.* Princeton, NJ: Princeton University Press.

Dublin, L., & Bunzel, B. (1933). *To be or not to be: A study in suicide.* New York: Harrison Smith and Robert Haas. Cited from https://babel.hathitrust.org/cgi/pt?id=mdp.39015004193903;view=1up;seq=202.

Freud, S. ([1901] (2018)). *The psychopathology of everyday living.* New Delhi: General Press.

Hartley, L. P. (1953). *The go-between.* London: Hamish Hamilton.

Hecht, J. M. (2013). *Stay: A history of suicide and the philosophies against it.* New Haven, CT: Yale University Press.

Lester, D., Sell, B., & Sell, K. (1980). *Suicide: A guide to information sources.* Detroit, MI: Gale Research Company.

Loeb Classical Library. (1931). *Book III, Exposition on stoicism* (Vol. XVII, 2nd revised ed., p. 281). Harvard University Press. Quote cited from http://penelope.uchicago.edu/Thayer/E/Roman/Texts/Cicero/de_Finibus/3*.html.

Minois, G. (2001). *History of suicide: Voluntary death in western culture.* Baltimore, MD: Johns Hopkins University Press.

Montesquieu in Battin, M.P. (2015). *The ethics of suicide: Historical sources*: 292–293. Oxford: Oxford University Press.

Murray, A. (1998, 2000). *Suicide in the middle ages: The violence against themselves* (Vol. 1). *Suicide in the middle ages: The curse of self-murder* (Vol. 2). Oxford: Oxford University Press.

Nordenfelt, L. (1997). The stoic conception of mental disorder: The case of Cicero. *Philosophy, Psychiatry, & Psychology, 4*(4), 285–291. Project MUSE, muse.jhu.edu/article/28206.

Perlin, S. (1975). *A handbook for the study of suicide.* New York: Oxford University Press.

Rosenbaum, R. (2001). *The secret parts of fortune: Three decades of intense investigations and edgy enthusiasm.* New York: Harper Perennial.

Rost, H. (1927). *Bibliographie des Selbstmord.* Augsburg: Hans U. Grabner.

Stannard, D. (1993). *American holocaust: Conquest of the new world.* London: Oxford University Press.

Szasz, T. (1974). *The secret sin.* New York: Anchor Books.

Wekstein, L. (1997). *A handbook of suicidology: Principles, problems and practice.* New York: Brunner/Mazel.

Chapter 5
The Aspirin Age

> *Society expects psychiatrists to prevent suicide. But this is*
> *unrealistic.*
>
> —Sidney Bloch [Emeritus professor of psychiatry,
> Melbourne University, author of *Understanding Troubled Minds*
> (2011).]
>
> *Depression: lowering of vitality or functional activity; dejection,*
> *as of mind.*
>
> —Webster's New International Dictionary

Abstract The jazz age after World War I, America's prohibition of alcohol, hangovers and the need for pain and anxiety relief; the age of psychoanalysis and psychology; the rapid progression from 'taking two Bex and a good lie-down' to antidepressants; the impact of the *DSM* on the medical profession.

Keywords Anxiety · Depression · Medical hegemony

The Aspirin Age (1965) is a book on American life between the two world wars, edited by Isobel Leighton, published in 1965. The 22 essays cover the chaotic years, the turbulence and pain in that anxious era, including the exploits of Izzy Einstein and Moe Smith as Prohibition detectives; the timely death of the crooked President Warren Gamaliel Harding, and the inertia of President Calvin Coolidge; the frightening violence of the Ku Klux Klan; the virulent antisemitic and pro-fascist radio broadcasts of Catholic Father Charles Coughlin; the Gene Tunney–Jack Dempsey heavyweight title fights; the Charles Lindbergh Jr. kidnapping; the stock market crash; the famous or infamous radio broadcast by actor Orson Welles of H. G. Wells' sci-fi tale *War of the Worlds*, which thousands of listeners thought was real, causing panic and total mayhem in New York; the New Deal [a series of public works projects]; the last days of Sacco and Vanzetti, two Italian-born American socialists dubiously convicted of armed robbery and sent to the electric chair amid public protests. In sum, a great

© Springer Nature Switzerland AG 2019   45
C. Tatz and S. Tatz, *The Sealed Box of Suicide*,
https://doi.org/10.1007/978-3-030-28159-5_5

depression. And in all that turmoil everyone needed an aspirin,[1] or aspirin plus. The frenetic inter-war years were not only an American affliction: Australia took on 'wowserism', a social attitude that sought to deprive the pleasures of those who were enjoying the 'sinful' life. The 'golden age' of psychoanalysis was to follow in the 1950s.

The saying 'take two aspirin and call me in the morning' originated from an era when doctors, in response to after-hours phone calls from patients unsure of what malady afflicted them, suggested the analgesic and a good rest. In Australia, you went to bed with one of two seductive choices—two 'Bex' or two 'Vincent's' (both a mix of powdered aspirin, phenacetin and caffeine), both available over the counter.

Antidepressants and anti-psychotics are today's aspirin; recommended and dispensed in increasing doses for a malady that, we believe, many medical practitioners simply do not understand, namely, suicidal behaviour. A 'solution' to suicide, a holy grail of *zero* deaths by self-intent, is in a yet-to-be discovered magic bullet, to be found in a genetic abnormality or biological anomaly. In the meantime, dispensing pills is one of the entrenched orthodoxies for depression, and by association, suicide prevention. In 2017–2018, Australia spent $A175 million on antidepressants under the Pharmaceutical Benefits Scheme (PBS). The other orthodoxy, consulting a clinical psychologist, cost the Medical Benefits Scheme (MBS) the sum of $A293 million.

5.1   Suicide and Depression

Suicide is deemed to be a consequence of a troubled mind, and the *troubled mind* belongs to specialists in the medical profession. The often-quoted statistic is that 90% of suicides are linked to depression; *ergo*, no person of right mind takes their own life; and who better to treat the troubled mind than those trained in psychiatric medicine? The axiom is that suicide is coupled with mental illness, a field of medicine under the auspice of psychiatrists (medical doctors with years of training), general practitioners and also psychologists who are not medically trained and unable to prescribe medication. (Our Chap. 12 discusses who is and who isn't trained, and the nature of professional training.)

The union of suicide and depression is entrenched. In *Shrinks* (2015), Jeffrey Lieberman's fascinating history of psychiatry and mental illness, he affirmed that 'the vast majority of people who commit suicide suffer from a mental illness, with depression being the most common' (Lieberman 2015: 214). [This dogma is now

---

[1]During World War II, youngsters in South Africa, the place of Colin Tatz's early years, drank three or four glasses of very effervescent Alka Seltzer in lieu of scarce Cokes or Pepsis, each tablet containing about 3.2 mg of acetylsalicylic acid. In the shortage of chewing gum, they used Aspergum, also with about 3.2 mg in each white rectangle. A lot of aspirin.

contested, as discussed elsewhere in this book.] Depression is a medical diagnosis treated primarily with antidepressants, a medication dispensed with alarming alacrity. It can also be treated with Cognitive Behavioural Therapy, short for talk therapy, and this approach is on the rise. Yet depression is a term commonly misused and misunderstood. The types of depression—major depression (clinical depression), melancholy, psychotic depression, antenatal and postnatal depression, bipolar disorder (manic depression), cyclothymic disorder, dysthymic disorder and seasonal affective disorder (SAD)—are opaque to the general public. *Depression* substitutes for a panoply of maladies, including what once were attributed to legitimate feelings of unhappiness, sadness, loss or grief. In the legal environment, the expressions 'mental illness' and 'depression' differ between jurisdictions and in interpretation. Defence lawyers frequently plead for mitigation as if depression—a condition the World Health Organization estimates affects about 300 million people world-wide—has a causal relationship with crime.

British investigative journalist Johann Hari's enlightening exploration of depression, *Lost Connections* (2018), is essential reading. To paraphrase his thesis, depression and anxiety are not necessarily the result of a troubled *mind* but of a troubled *world*, where individuals have lost their connections to activities and associations that create a more hopeful present and future. It is not a chemical imbalance that renders millions depressed; it is an imbalance in how we live, socially and spiritually. Depression, Hari persuasively demonstrated, is caused by biological, psychological and social factors, except the psychological and social are pushed asunder by the medical profession and pharmaceutical industry. The evidence for medication as *the* treatment doesn't add up. In the world Hari has experienced, human beings are not 'a machine with broken parts … [we] are an animal whose needs are not being met'. These needs encompass a sense of community, relations with other people; meaningful (not junk) values; learning that happiness isn't derived from money or consumerism; engaging in work that is secure, valid and meaningful; status and respect; and connections to the natural world (Hari 2018: 256–257).

Recognising social and psychological connections—as in emotions, feelings and pain—as factors in suicide was raised by Edwin Shneidman, founder of the Los Angeles Suicide Prevention Center, over 50 years ago. Shneidman, credited with the term 'psychological autopsy', viewed suicide as fundamentally, but not always, about psychological pain:

> Suicide is caused by psychache … the hurt, anguish, soreness, aching, psychological pain in the psyche, the mind. It is intrinsically psychological – the pain of excessively felt shame, or guilt, or humiliation. When it occurs, its reality is introspectively undeniable. Suicide occurs when the psychache is deemed by that person to be unbearable. This means that suicide also has to do with different individual thresholds for enduring psychological pain. (Shneidman and Farberow 1965)

Writing half a century ago, Shneidman understood that 'the essential nature of suicides is not clearly understood. It is not a single disease entity', something the French physician Esquirol told us in the nineteenth century.

By coupling suicide and mental illness under the medical umbrella, it *is* all but considered a single disease entity. Schwartz-Lifshitz et al. (2012), for example, insisted that:

> More than half of all clinically depressed persons have suicidal ideation and major depression disorder, and bipolar disorders are the psychiatric disorders most often associated with suicide. Some symptoms of depression have been identified as particularly important in risk for suicidal behaviour: hopelessness, feelings of guilt, loss of interest, insomnia, and low self esteem. (Schwartz-Lifshitz et al. 2012)

The literature abounds with similar links between suicide and depression. Missing is the explicit acknowledgment that a great many millions of people with depression do *not* suicide or self-harm. This judgment is so ingrained that medical experts can succumb to hindsight bias, moulding the troubled mind concept around suicides regardless of other possibilities. Post-mortem, they look for depression, insights into suicidal ideation or behaviour, expressions of intent or mental illness. [Below we refer to recent research in Sydney showing that suiciders who saw medical professionals a month before they took their lives gave no indications of 'ideation'.]

A Handbook for the Study of Suicide (Perlin 1975) is atypical of the entrenched belief that suicide must derive from mental illness. In the chapter titled *Biology*, Solomon Snyder understandably pondered 'if biological studies may be relevant in any way to mental illness' and later asks if the commonly postulated 'mechanism' is that those who take their own lives 'have lost a zest for living' (in Perlin 1975: 114–115). What comes next, however, is a delve into the science of neurotransmitter specific tracts in the brain and norepinephrine metabolisms and the study of 'reward centres'. Snyder's conclusion was to wonder if the 'catecholamine hypothesis' may be right, and thus open up the study of chemical agents in treating mental illness. Texts and academic medical papers of this ilk frustrate the layperson. We flounder in the small fonts describing dysfunctions in the central noradrenergic system that may account for mental illnesses that become suicides, or abnormalities of serotonergic mechanism, or the point where the amygdala receives a signal from the prefrontal cortex. The neurobiology of suicide has us reaching for medical textbooks and online search engines to understand why a deficit or surplus of this or that component of the mind accounts for suicide. [As we discuss in Chap. 6, to which of the 36 categories of suicide would such analyses be applicable, or useful?]

Probing the cranium in search of the exact chemical imbalance or dysfunctions in the serotonergic system may, hopefully, provide some medical outcomes to reduce suicides. While we await this scientific breakthrough, we take issue that hopelessness, feelings of guilt, loss of interest in aspects of life, insomnia, low self-esteem, loneliness, shame, alienation, racism, poverty, bullying, stigmatising or being embedded in a world of helplessness can be 'cured' by medication adjusting the chemical imbalances. As we discuss in Chap. 12 on professionals, the high rate of suicide among physicians (anaesthetists and psychiatrists in particular) is not all that often attributed to 'chemical imbalances'. Nonetheless, it is to pharmacology and medication that society turns, even when mounting evidence indicates medication can only be partially effective.

5.2   Suicide and the Diagnostic and Statistical Manual of Mental Disorders (DSM)

Jeffrey Lieberman defined the *DSM* as the 'bible of psychiatry'. Like the scriptures, proclaimed as gospel by people of faith, Lieberman nominated the *DSM* as 'the most influential book written in the past century'. The *DSM* is a 'career manual' for psychiatrists; it 'dictates' payments; it is referenced in compensation claims; court cases are decided on a defendant's mental abilities apropos the *DSM*. Education systems are constructed according to it; funding and research is 'granted or denied' based on its diagnostic criteria; and billions of dollars of pharmaceutical research stem from the *DSM*. The *DSM*, said Lieberman, has 'unparalleled medical influence over society' (Lieberman 2015: 87).

For patients, a diagnosis of depression or other mental illnesses follows the ticking of appropriate *DSM* boxes. It perpetuates the belief that manifestations of mental illness are chronic lifetime conditions, to be treated by psychopharmaceuticals. Before *DSM-5* was released in 2013, proposals were afoot for suicide to be included, as *New Scientist* revealed:

> The team behind the fifth edition of the *Diagnostic Standards Manual* (*DSM-5*) … considered a proposal to have 'suicide behaviour disorder' listed as a distinct diagnosis. It was ultimately put on probation: put into a list of topics deemed to require further research for possible inclusion in future *DSM* revisions. Another argument for linking suicidal people together under a single diagnosis is that it could spur research into the neurological and genetic factors they have in common. This could allow psychiatrists to better predict someone's suicide risk, and even lead to treatments that stop suicidal feelings. (Reardon 2013)

Suicidal behaviour may yet end up in the *DSM*. There are those in the psychiatric profession advocating for a clearly delineated criterion. The reasons *not* to include suicide on the *DSM* are powerful. This medical gospel has a contentious history of labelling and defining medical conditions, as Scully (2004) pointed out in her paper on diseases: 'It might not be easy to articulate what a disease is, but we like to think we would at least all know when we see one. Unfortunately, this is problematic as well. Notions of health are highly context-dependent, as human diseases only exist in relation to people, and people live in varied cultural contexts'. The author cited homosexuality as an example: in the nineteenth century, it was reclassified as 'a state' as opposed to an 'act'. Early in the twentieth century, homosexuality became 'an endocrine disturbance requiring hormone treatment' before being categorised 'as an organic mental disorder treatable by electroshock and sometimes neurosurgery'.

The *DSM*, wrote British psychiatrist Burton (2015), has 'followed in a long tradition in medicine and psychiatry, which in the nineteenth century appropriated homosexuality from the church and, in an élan of enlightenment, transformed it from sin to mental disorder'. At the American Psychiatric Association (APA) convention in 1973, APA members actually voted on 'whether they believed homosexuality to be a mental disorder. While 5854 psychiatrists voted to remove homosexuality from the *DSM*, a staggering 3810 psychiatrists voted to retain it' (Burton 2015). It took 14 more years before the *DSM* finally removed homosexuality from its books. Including suicidal behaviour disorder in the *DSM*, with accompanying guidelines for medical practitioners in prediction and prevention, would further entrench the act of ending one's life prematurely as a diagnosable illness. The process of medicalisation converts a human emotion, action or response into one requiring medical treatment, entrenching health care providers as the major, even the only, deliverers of 'help'. (Teachers, priests, social workers, counsellors, friends, family elders have roles to play in situations of emotional distress.)

The idea that suicide should be considered a disease or condition is something more than merely contentious. Is suicidality one attempt, two 'goes' or a half dozen; or is it the expression of the desire to kill oneself? Who knows how many human beings throughout history have thoughts of suicide? Statistics offer limited insight: in 2013, an estimated 9.3 million American adults (3.9%) aged 18 or older had serious thoughts of suicide in the previous year, a percentage that remained stable between 2008 and 2013.[2] A 2017 study in the UK found an appreciably higher per cent of White people—21.6%—reported having a suicidal thought at some stage in their lives.[3] Would over 9 million Americans be classified, under a *DSM* diagnosis, as suicidal? If it is not normal to have suicidal thoughts, it most certainly isn't abnormal. Passing thoughts of ending one's life are a social fact in human history, common, oftentimes during intense moments of shame, guilt, loss or a reaction to oppressive situations. As an individual's circumstances change, so too does behaviour and response. Suicidal behaviour, even expressed, is not necessarily a symptom of mental illness, nor should it be a definition of a medical disorder; it may be a momentary reaction to events, or a way of gaining attention. How a *DSM* or medical criteria differentiates between having and acting on these thoughts is quite unclear.

Suicide behaviours, including attempts, can be situational, perhaps fleeting. Even reoccurring attempts may be more a cry for help than a clinical condition. We were told a story of a woman who appeared at a major emergency department every weekend, screaming hysterically and by all indications, mentally unwell and possibly suicidal. Medical interventions did not prevent her from returning in a state that

---

[2]Results from the 2013 National Survey on Drug Use and Health: Mental Health Findings. U.S. Department of Health and Human Services, Substance Abuse and Mental Health Services Administration Center for Behavioral Health Statistics and Quality. https://www.samhsa.gov/data/sites/default/files/NSDUHresultsPDFWHTML2013/Web/NSDUHresults2013.pdf.

[3]'Adults reporting suicidal thoughts, attempts and self-harm', See: www.ethnicity-facts-figures.service.gov.uk/health/physical-and-mental-health/adults-reporting-suicidal-thoughts-attempts-and-self-harm/latest.

alarmed triage staff and those waiting for emergency medical care. Eventually, the hospital found a solution. A room was set up with comfortable sofa, tea and coffee, candles and soothing music. When the highly distressed woman next appeared, they welcomed her warmly and invited her to sit with the medical staff and relax with a cup of tea. After much talking, they discovered she was desperately lonely, and the hospital was the only place where she interacted. Her near-suicidal hysteria was indeed a cry for attention. Hospital staff connected her with a women's support group and never saw her again. 'Social prescribing' is the name given to this approach. It doesn't flourish, mental health policy expert Dr. Sebastian Rosenberg told us, because of the lack of professional health care training.

5.3   The Medical Domination of Suicide

'The starting point in treating the suicidal person', wrote emeritus professor of psychiatry Bloch (2011: 255) 'is seen so differently by psychiatrists and patients'. The concept of suicide, a 'voluntary rejection of the value of life', was, in Bloch's words, a threat to psychiatrists' convictions. [Baechler pointed out that for doctors and psychiatrists every death is a defeat (Baechler 1979: 24).] In his refreshing examination of mental illness, Bloch sought explanations for suicide among medical practitioners (psychiatrists in particular), retelling his own experience of plunging into such depression that he too 'harboured suicidal thoughts'. Bloch, perhaps an outlier in his field, recognised that 'psychiatrists' ability to predict who will kill themselves is limited and is likely to remain so', but they 'do what they can to reduce the rate'. He concluded that we 'have not reached the point at which mental health and related social services are sufficiently developed to meet the population's needs' (Bloch 2011: 272).

Bloch's acknowledgment of the limitations of psychiatry was confirmed by a landmark study by the University of New South Wales in 2019. This research revealed that the majority of people who suicided had denied expressing suicidal thoughts when questioned by their physician in the weeks and months prior to their suicide. The analysis undertaken by clinical psychiatrist Professor Matthew Large challenged the notion that psychiatrists can predict with any certainty a patient's likelihood of committing suicide (Carroll 2019). The data review, compiled from 70 studies of suicidal thoughts, concluded that 'as a stand-alone test, only 1.7% of people with suicidal ideas died by suicide. About 60% of people who died by suicide had denied having suicidal thoughts when asked by a psychiatrist or GP'. As Large explained, 'this study proves we can no longer ration psychiatric care based on the presence of suicidal thoughts alone'. Team researcher Catherine McHugh said that medical practitioners 'sometimes rely on what is known as suicidal ideation—being preoccupied with thoughts and planning suicide—as a crucial test for short-term suicide risk, and it has been argued it could form part of a screening test for suicide. Our results show that this is not in the best interests of patients'.

The meta-analysis cited above may be just one study; nonetheless, it is to medical practitioners and psychiatrists that many in the population and most politicians look for a *solution* to suicide and the chimera of zero suicide. In Australia, the conservative government has vowed to pursue 'an obsessive goal of towards zero suicides'; their mechanism for achieving this is to appoint a special adviser on mental health and increase access to psychologist sessions (McCauley 2019).

Contrasting Bloch's honest assessment of psychiatry's limitations, another leading Australian psychiatrist told us that *all* suicides are the result of mental illness, *ipso facto*, psychiatry and mental health professionals must be at the vanguard of managing this condition, disorder, public health problem or whatever is the current nomenclature that casts suicide within the domain of biomedicine. Psychiatrists (and to a lesser extent psychologists and GPs) are said to be highly trained in diagnosing and treating mental illness. Their role is to explain, to understand and categorise disorders, then provide appropriate treatments. Their resource is their training, mostly devoid of any social science findings, with the *DSM* providing social contexts beyond the mainstream. These social contexts may include stable and secure housing, meaningful employment, peer support, relationships, access to transport and services, education; and even connections to sport, religion, the arts, nature. In discussions with psychiatrists, we have been told it is mistaken ideology that allows non-psychiatrists leadership roles in mental health and suicide; that housing, employment and financial stress are matters addressed *after* medication and psychiatric treatments. Their most effective and efficient way to treat people who are suicidal is 'medical treatment', meaning medication and hospitalisation.

Psychiatry is not our target. We both engage with psychiatrists professionally, personally, socially, as colleagues and consultants. For once the cliché 'some of my best friends...' (are psychiatrists) is appropriate. Diagnosis, classification, and pharmacology in *aspects* of suicide prevention are not in dispute. Many people with severe and ongoing mental illness undoubtedly benefit from psychiatric care, as psychiatrists are able to intercede to prevent suicides in individual cases. Our curiosity lies in the dominance of mainstream mental health medication in suicide as the dominant and sometimes dogmatic *solution.* We question whether clinicians can prevent suicide using the same strategies and investigations into the neurobiology of suicide. An analogy with the war on drugs comes to mind. Coincidentally, the war on drugs began around the same time suicide preventions embarked on their mission. To date, no country, no amount of expenditure, no army (state or private), no death penalty or jail time has made any substantial impact on personal illicit drug use, although in defined regions and jurisdictions illicit drug use has been reduced, often through implementing harsh penalties. However, in Portugal, the problem has been managed effectively through radical legislative reforms that position personal drug use as a health, not a criminal justice issue. The suicide analogy with the campaign to prevent illegal drug use is valid. Put simply, medication and medicalisation work in part, in certain circumstances, among some cohorts. Medication has not, and is unlikely to, *prevent* suicides.[4] The drugs may well defer, delay or deflect, but there is not sufficient evidence that they will stop the phenomenon of self-death.

5.4 Power Imbalances

Health systems are constructed with inbuilt power imbalances. This is particularly evident in situations where individuals are rendered powerless or unable to provide voice, such as residential aged care facilities, those with intellectual disabilities and people deemed 'mad' or suicidal. Those with lived experience of mental illness are given the designation 'consumers'. What they are consuming is not entirely evident, although they are almost always referred to as *suffering* a mental illness (whereas those with cancer bravely *battle* their disease). Language reinforces stigma—the suicidal person *suffered* a mental illness as if victims of an evil disease, a curse or 'something' that somehow invaded them. Mental health consumers say power imbalance can prove an obstacle to their recovery and resilience. Patients consult psychiatrists, psychologists or general practitioners and, based on the *DSM* or another clinical assessment tool, are given a diagnosis, most often accompanied by a prescription for antidepressant medication.

Professor Diana Rose is but one advocate challenging the power relationship and its impact. Rose is in a unique position to defy the status quo; she is a *consumer,* Professor of User-Led Research, and co-director of the Institute of Psychiatry, Psychology and Neuroscience's Service User Research Enterprise at King's College in London. Presenting at a mental health conference in Melbourne in 2018, her challenging keynote address questioned medical hegemony on mental health (and by extension, suicide), suggesting mainstream research is neither value-free nor neutral, and that 'research is not the only way of creating knowledge'.

Although Rose was referring to mental health, her rationalisation is applicable to suicide:

> You might not think research involves a power dynamic but it does, especially in mental health. Most researchers are also clinicians and the people they're doing the research on are patients. That clinician/patient dynamic is replicated in the research setting. If the methodology is fixed, you can have very little influence. If you can't change the way the information is collected, you can't change the way it's analysed. All you can do is tinker around the edges.

As Rose explained, 'User-led research promotes a different way of listening to those in distress and so figuring what it means. Mainstream research often doesn't lis-

---

[4]A Swedish study, 'Antidepressant medication and suicide in Sweden', by Carlsten et al. (2001), has shown a correlation between antidepressants and lowered suicide rates. Cited at: https://onlinelibrary.wiley.com/doi/abs/10.1002/pds.618.

ten at all'. For this pioneering mental health researcher, the imbalance allows health systems to be driven by clinicians seeking data and outcome measures. Tellingly, Rose summed up the current approach this way: 'I don't mean you shouldn't have this, but you shouldn't just have this'. The Banfield et al. study (2012) on health consumers' priorities concluded that participants reflect an interest in a holistic approach to mental health research, one that examines the influences of everyday life and psychosocial influences both on the development and on the management of these disorders. Their focus was on research that explores individualised care and the active role that consumers can play in their own care.

Before psychiatrists and mental health practitioners sharpen their figurative swords and send invitations to the lynch mob, they should ponder the exposition we have adapted from Rose and others. Psychiatry is not being disabused. But psychiatry and the medical profession constitute a power imbalance. Suicide is deemed a medical condition *they* diagnose and they treat persons using *their* diagnostic tools and medications *they* prescribe. The patient/client/consumer is all too often disenfranchised from engaging in co-design of diagnosis or treatment. In this sense, co-design refers to the way patients are involved in the design process and how they work with physicians to understand their met and unmet needs. Psychiatric care should engage their patients in some co-designed relationship where their goals and outcomes are identified. But too often those assessed as suicidal, or at risk, have no input into the diagnostic tools used or the assessments made. The relationship between doctor and patient is generally one of subservience; you are diagnosed, labelled, and in most cases medicated, a situation experienced in others aspects of health care.

As we pondered why psychiatrists sit atop the medico pyramid in predicting and preventing suicide, along came *Pharmacy Times* (Marotta 2018). In a provocatively titled article, '5 Ways Pharmacists Can Help Prevent Suicide', it informed readers that 'pharmacists are ideally suited' to suicide prevention due to their 'frequent interactions with patients' and their 'unique position' in dispensing 'mental health medications such as antidepressants'. The medicalisation of suicide and dispensing of medications continues apace.

5.5   The Magic Pill

Statistics date quickly. Data available today will be superseded tomorrow. What we know is that currently Australia is credited with one of the highest rates of antidepressant use in the world, a rate that has more than doubled since 2000. About 10% of adult Australians are using antidepressants, 'despite evidence showing that the effectiveness of these medications is lower than previously thought'. World-wide, prescriptions for antidepressants are increasing. The American rate for consuming these pills is around 13%. Davey and Chanen (2016) explained the increase in antidepressant use as a consequence of the 1980 *DSM-III*, which extended the diagnostic interpretation of depression, and the arrival of SSRIs (selective serotonin reuptake inhibitors) two years later, events that ensured the 'cultural phenomenon that encouraged us to think of depression as resulting from a chemical imbalance that could be corrected' (Davey and Chanen 2016).

The evidence that antidepressants and anti-psychotic medications reduce suicide is contentious. As non-clinicians, we must accept reports and published papers indicating certain medications are effective among selected cohorts, and new advances in anti-psychotic medications are reducing severe side effects and improving patient outcomes. Yet we weigh this against the alternative—that in lieu of known treatments or preventions, the biomedical reaction to patients who may be suicidal or experience mental illness is to medicate. The medical options are limited—antidepressants, anti-psychotic medications, anti-anxiety medications—typically prescribed for patients expressing suicidal thoughts or 'symptoms', a term we often encounter but still do not understand.

Evidence is now pointing to another, counter outcome, one that questions medication as a frontline treatment. In conducting our research, we read peer-reviewed articles and news reports examining the relationship between antidepressant medication and suicide (as in the Swedish study cited above). Hundreds of approved medications now nominate suicidal symptoms as side effects (as we discussed earlier in the Prozac court case). Warnings do not indicate likelihood or responsibility, however, the possibility that so many medications *may* impact on suicidal behaviour should alarm doctors enough to be cautious in prescribing antidepressant as a frontline treatment for mental illness and suicide prevention.

This quest for that elusive cure-all should fill research grants and pharmaceutical company's budgets, yet paradoxically there is an under-investment. The Pharmaceutical Research and Manufacturers of America trade group reported in 2018 that 'drugmakers have 140 therapies in development targeting mental health issues, including 39 aimed at depression' yet the pharmaceutical industry is working on about 1100 experimental cancer drugs, which not surprisingly are sold at higher prices (Steenhuysen 2018).

These modern-day evangelists cite positive outcomes in individual cases as *the* wonder cure. The underlying causes of suicide are scantily noted in passing. The holy grail remains a biological intervention, the magic pill that mutes suicidal thoughts, behaviours and actions. For researcher Moises Velasquez-Manoff (2018), Ketamine was the magic treatment that 'can halt suicidal thoughts almost immediately'. Psychiatrists, he wrote, desperately need such 'new treatment options. In the USA, pharmaceutical companies and self-named 'clinics' are scrambling on to the Ketamine train, despite negligible evidence regarding its efficacy. These clinics are charging up to $1000 for 'treatments' despite the absence of clinical data or published evidence. Jeffrey Lieberman is alarmed; patients are 'getting treatments they may not need or that don't work, or they're getting more than they needed … [with Ketamine] people are getting fleeced' (Thielking 2018). Ketamine does not address fundamental problems in society or individual circumstances.

Ketamine is not alone. Discussing Shneidman's work on suicide, New York psychiatrist Anne Skomorowsky (2017) pondered if mental pain (psychache) can be treated like physical pain to reduce suicide: it too has a neurobiological process which can be ameliorated through low doses of opioids. Skomorowsky made a telling point: currently 'there are no medications to quickly relieve suicidal thoughts' as antidepressants take months to kick in. Many psychiatrists, she said, are now believing Schneidman's view that 'depression and suicidal ideation are separate conditions'. Where we depart from the Skomorowskys of this world is her faith in 'a medication that specifically targets suicidal ideation', such as the opioid buprenorphine.

In treating mental health, we hear of the importance of multi-disciplinary, multi-agency team approaches as the most effective (and efficient) way to help people. Led by a psychiatrist or GP, this approach recognises that people's well-being can only be improved if they are surrounded by a suite of supports: medical, social and economic. *Wrap-around services* is the buzz word. Not surprisingly, this concept is yet to be universally accepted; the resisters are, unsurprisingly, those with entrenched faith in the *DSM*. To us, a multi-agency approach seems eminently logical in suicide alleviation and deflection.

5.6   Novel Ideas

It may well be time to resurrect two fine novels by Aldous Huxley, both published in the aspirin age: *Brave New World* (BNW), published in 1932—rated in the top 100 best novels of all time—is a dystopian satire, forecasting the age of genetics, genetic modifications, the era of designer babies. It tells of a society of manufactured humans, arranged in a hierarchy of intelligence, with alpha plus males at the top and muscular, gorilla-like epsilons at the bottom as a slave class. But whatever the mental capacities of new world members, they all need aspirin, what Huxley called 'soma': a government-issue drug to ease pain, to alleviate discomfort, embarrassment, sadness or anger, to enhance joy and feelings of well-being. Soma has been upgraded to Prozac. In a later novel, *After Many a Summer* (1939), Huxley flays materialism, consumerism and narcissism in particular—the hyper-concerns about health, longer life, even everlasting life. His billionaire protagonist seeks the royal jelly, the secret of good health, [good skin, good looks, nice internal rhythms] and immortality, only to discover that evolution can work backwards and life as a rich ape-man isn't fun.

To what purpose we don't know, but research has found that for better or for worse, in sickness and in health, female starlings fed with Prozac are less attentive to male birds and are less likely to mate. And in the case of crabs, crustaceans fed on the drug are five times more likely to spend time in the light than those that are off the drug and lurk in the murk.

References

Banfield, M. A., Barney, L. J., Griffiths, K. M., & Christensen, H. M. (2012). *Australian mental health consumers priorities for research: Qualitative findings from the SCOPE for Research project*. Australian Primary Health Care Research Institute. Cited at: https://onlinelibrary.wiley.com/doi/full/10.1111/j.1369-7625.2011.00763.x.

Baechler, J. (1979). *Suicides*. New York Basic Books.

Bloch, S. (2011). *Understanding troubled minds*. Melbourne: Melbourne University.

Burton, N. (2015, September 18). When homosexuality stopped being a mental disorder. *Psychology Today*. Cited at: https://www.psychologytoday.com/us/blog/hide-and-seek/201509/when-homosexuality-stopped-being-mental-disorder.

Carlsten, A., Waern, M., Ekedahl A., & Ranstam, J. (2001). Antidepressant medication and suicide in Sweden. Cited at: https://onlinelibrary.wiley.com/doi/abs/10.1002/pds.618.

Carroll, L. (2019). Suicidal thoughts not a reliable warning of suicide. *NSWU Newsroom* (media release). https://newsroom.unsw.edu.au/news/health/suicidal-thoughts-not-reliable-warning-suicide.

Davey, C. G., & Andrew, C. (2016). The unfulfilled promise of the antidepressant medications. *Medical Journal of Australia, 204*(9): 348–350. https://doi.org/10.5694/mja16.00194. Published online: 16 May. Google: https://www.ncbi.nlm.nih.gov/pmc/articles/PMC1256136/pdf/amjphnation00153-0023.pdf.

Hari, J. (2018). *Lost connections: Uncovering the causes of depression—and unexpected solutions*. London: Bloomsbury Circus.

Huxley, A. (1932). *Brave new world*. London: Chatto & Windus.

Huxley, A. (1939). *After many a summer*. London: Chatto & Windus.

Leighton, I. (1965). *The aspirin age: 1919–1941*. New York: Simon and Schuster.

Lieberman, J. (2015). *Shrinks: The untold story of psychiatry*. New York: Little, Brown Company.

Marotta, R. (2018, June 8). 5 ways pharmacists can help prevent suicide. *Pharmacy Times*.

McCauley, D. (2019, June 1). Hunt pledges action on youth suicide. *The Age*.

Oquendo, M., & Baca-Garcia, E. (2014, June). Suicidal behavior disorder as a diagnostic entity in the DSM-5 classification system: Advantages outweigh limitations. *World Psychiatry, 13*(2), 128–130. Cited at: https://www.ncbi.nlm.nih.gov/pmc/articles/PMC4102277.

Perlin, S. (1975). *A handbook for the study of suicide*. New York: Oxford University Press.

Reardon, S. (2013, May 7). Suicidal behaviour is a disease, psychiatrists argue. *New Scientist*. Cited at: www.newscientist.com/article/dn23566-suicidal-behaviour-is-a-disease-psychiatrists-argue/.

Schwartz-Lifshitz, M., Zalsman, G., Giner, L., et al. (2012) Can we really prevent suicide? *Current Psychiatry Reports, 14*, 624. Cited at: https://link.springer.com/article/10.1007/s11920-012-0318-3.

Scully, J. L. (2004, July). What is a disease? *EMBO Reports, 5*(7), 650–653. https://doi.org/10.1038/sj.embor.7400195. PMCID: PMC1299105. PMID: 15229637 in Science and Society. See: www.ncbi.nlm.nih.gov/pmc/articles/PMC1299105/.

Shneidman, E. S., & Farberow, N. L. (1965). *The Los Angeles suicide prevention center: A demonstration of public health feasibilities*. https://www.ncbi.nlm.nih.gov/pmc/articles/PMC1256136/pdf/amjphnation00153-0023.pdf.

Skomorowsky, A. (2017). How to prevent suicide with an opioid. *Scientific American Mind, 28*, 70–73. Published online: 8 July 2017. Cited at: https://www.scientificamerican.com/article/how-to-prevent-suicide-with-an-opioid/.

Steenhuysen, J. (2018, 9 June). Rise in U.S. suicides highlights need for new depression drugs. *Reuters*. Cited at: https://www.reuters.com/article/us-health-suicide-drugs/rise-in-us-suicides-highlights-need-for-new-depression-drugs-idUSKCN1J42TO.

Thielking, M. (2018). Ketamine gives hope to patients with severe depression. But some clinics stray from the science and hype its benefits. Cited at: https://www.statnews.com/2018/09/24/ketamine-clinics-severe-depression-treatment/.

Velasquez-Manoff, M. (2018, November 30). Can we stop suicides? *New York Times*.

Chapter 6
Diverse Suicides

There comes a time when you look into the mirror and you realise that what you see is all that you will ever be. And then you accept it. Or you kill yourself. Or you stop looking in mirrors.

—Tennessee Williams [American playwright, 1911–1983]

That's the thing about suicide. Try as you might to remember how a person lived his life, you always end up thinking about how he ended it.

—Anderson Cooper [American journalist and author. Quoted from CNN International extract of 'My brother's suicide', *Details Magazine*, September 2003]

Abstract Why suicide is not a single or a singular behaviour; the many categories of suicide; the need for prevention strategists to target the disparate suicides, to differentiate the kinds that can possibly be prevented from those that cannot be. Similarly, an examination of suicide methods and access to them.

Keywords Suicide categories · Methods · Access to modes

After heart disease, cancer is the second-ranked cause of death, at least in the West. Medicine distinguishes at least a hundred forms of cancer, ranging from acute lymphoblastic leukaemia at the top of the alphabet to intraocular melanoma midway and young adult cancer at the tail of the list. Specialist physicians, dedicated wards and nurses and highly specific chemicals treat these distinguishable forms of what the American oncologist Siddhartha Mukherjee calls 'the emperor of all maladies' (2010). Suicide is nowhere near that high in the death ranking, and while it is a social symptom rather than a disease, why is it always presented as a single phenomenon?

We counted 36 differing categories of suicide. Some are quite evident, others are theoretical, several are speculative and a few are culture-specific. But attempts to prevent, reduce or treat the behaviour among the still living need to make the essential distinctions between them, however broadly. Some medical personnel may do just that, but we know of no prevention agency that thinks of suicide as other than a one-headed enemy to be eliminated.

Categorisation after the event will also have its uses. While post-mortem unravelling of suicide causation is hardly a science, even with the services of a skilled forensic anthropologist, the deceased's profile may well have value in the approach to relatives and close friends.

It cannot be said that we lack a literature on the diverse categories of suicide. Rather, it must be concluded that those who deal with the subject don't seem to bother with the writings of the elders. Who but sociology undergraduates read Durkheim's *Le suicide* published 122 years ago? Or Jean Baechler's *Suicides* of 45 years ago? Durkheim gave us the categories of egoistic suicide, altruistic suicide, fatalistic suicide and anomic suicide. Looked at carefully, his broad classifications are hardly *passé*. And, his categories were based essentially on human relationships within a society, not chemical interactions in the brain. (We note that very few of the seminal books on suicide have been written by psychiatrists; two or three by psychologists, yes, but in the main, it is the philosophers and the sociologists who have communicated and conveyed systematic and integrated analysis of the phenomenon.)

Sociologists have provided useful broad genres or styles of motivation for suicide. The Italian Marzio Barbagli divided suicide into those who commit the act *for* selves or *for* others and those who do it as a form of revenge *against* others (Barbagli 2015). Our history chapter notes Eastern societies where revenge—in the shape of a suicider's ghost haunting the doorstep of an oppressor—was common. From France's Baechler, we have a strangely named quartet: *escapist* (flight, grief and punishment); *oblative* (sacrifice and transfiguration), the latter akin to Jean Améry's exit from physical life to that other place called death; *ludic* (the ordeal, the gambling with one's life); and *aggressive* (crime, vengeance, blackmail and appealing, as in anthropologist Emanuel Marx below) (Baechler 1975). The American Jack Douglas wrote about *escape*, *revenge* and *sympathy* genres (Douglas 1967).

As to categories within these genres, we have the invaluable framework of the eminent psychopathologist Louis Wekstein whose *Handbook of Suicidology* sets out his variations and classifications of suicide behaviour (Wekstein 1979). His categories were certainly diverse, covering suicide gestures, ambivalent suicide attempts, serious suicide attempts and completed suicides. His typology immediately suggested that differing approaches are needed for diverse suicide types. In Chap. 7, we touch on the three categories presented by historians Miller and Miller (1992, 1999): *despairing, altruistic* and *defiant suicide*. Yet prevention agencies, at least in Australia, make little or no effort to address these disparities: their target is both intervention and prevention, two different actions, and in the latter case, there is no obvious effort to differentiate between genres or kinds of suicide. At best, that is consonant with the adamantine view of suicide as mental illness: thus, so the formula goes, treat the illness and the suicide will go away. Durkheim, Wekstein, the Millers and others have rightly shown that there are several manners of suicide categories that have nothing to do with mental illness. And, there are suicides that are simply not amenable to therapies of any kind. To Durkheim's four, we list Wekstein's 11 categories, the Millers' two others, and in addition to one of Durkheim's, we suggest another 19 categories for consideration.

6.1 Thirty-Six Categories

Egoistic suicide, wrote Durkheim, occurs when a person becomes socially isolated or feels that they have no place in the society. *Alienation* is a good enough synonym for that sense of not belonging. In 1908, the German sociologist Georg Simmel (1858–1918) wrote a powerful essay entitled 'The Stranger' in which he defined this social category of person—not the outsider but the socially alienated person who is cut off by the mainstream society (Simmel 1908). Social isolation has certainly increased with the advent of gadgetry and computer technology, as discussed below.

Altruistic suicide for Durkheim is not quite the way we see this category. For him, an individual who lives in a highly regulated society and who is well integrated will commit suicide in certain circumstances, as in Japanese and Hindu customs—what we call, below, *honour suicide* or *sacrificial suicide*. *Altruistic suicide* is also a form of sacrifice on behalf of others. In Chap. 7, we discuss the ways in which Armenian grandmothers sent on death marches by the Turks in World War I would stay behind, certain to die, in order not to hold up mothers and grandchildren being coerced along the way to Syria.

There is another facet of altruism—those 26,513 men and women honoured by Israel as Righteous Gentiles, or the Righteous Among the Nations, that is, non-Jews who hid Jews for no reward and at risk to their lives and property during World War II. They hid Jews in their homes and farms in seemingly impossible circumstances, somehow obtained extra food for them during rationing and scarcity, furnished them with false papers, smuggled them to safety or rescued Jewish children in imaginative ways. These actions were met with summary execution of the 'perpetrator' and their immediate family. Many were so killed for their efforts; and, they knew that their survival possibility was unrealistic.

Fatalistic suicide, stated Durkheim, is a result of a pervasive oppression, or a feeling that such is the case—an existential dilemma perhaps from which death is the best escape mechanism. Some writers have cited slavery as a classic case of this type of self-inflicted death. Snyder's work (2010, 2015) on the 1803 suicides of Igbo slaves from Nigeria who, after revolting against the slaver boat crew, drowned themselves collectively when put ashore in America's Georgia. Snyder wrote graphically about the efforts of slavers to stop their 'cargo' from jumping overboard, resorting to all manner of devices and netting to stop them jumping. Slave crews also invented a ghastly metal device, called the *speculum oris*, designed specifically to force-feed slaves who went on hunger strikes in protest at their mistreatment. One might consider their end to this suffering as *despairing suicide* (of which more appears below).

Fatalistic suicide of this (physically entrapped) kind is easier to comprehend than the circumstance of one who feels oppressed or suffocated by society, or 'the system'. The latter has at times been called *anomic* or *existential suicide* by several analysts, especially Camus (1955) and Améry (1999). There are, certainly, those people who 'have had enough' of what they see as the hypocrisy and the meaninglessness of life, imprecise but comprehensible emotions. There is a degree of understanding about physical extremes, whether it is a slavery ship, a terrible prison system or, where in Australia, for example, asylum-seekers have been placed in long-term and unrelenting detention on tiny Nauru in the Pacific and on Manus Island in Papua New Guinea in an agreement with those island governments. There, children as young as 10 years old have been attempting suicide. Categorisation is often a difficult exercise, but one might as easily call this *despairing suicide*. The Millers (1992, 1999) used this term about Armenian women who faced lives of sexual slavery under the Turks in World War I.[1]

How do preventionists deal with this behaviour? Corrective and prison services, certainly in Australia, have installed every conceivable surveillance system of 'suicide watch'—as much to protect lives as institutional reputations. The Aboriginal Deaths in Custody Royal Commission of 1991 still hovers heavily over corrective service institutions. No one wants a repeat of those tough and very public interrogations.[2] But what of those unconfined? Some in the categories mentioned above talk, write, behave oddly, 'act up', 'slash up', 'seek attention', take to their beds or to reclusiveness, and can be assisted in several ways. A great many appear to give no overt signs, leaving relatives and friends as much shocked and bewildered as sad.

Anomic suicide, said the French sociologist, occurs where a society fails to regulate its members, typically in modern industrial societies. One could well add the haphazard suburban growth of cities and the lack of infrastructure when immigration policies don't take account of incoming numbers of migrants and their needs. Australia is not alone in failing to accommodate migrant population growth.

Astonishment usually greets the suicides of pop musicians and sportspeople—who are believed to 'have everything'. *Celebrity suicide* is accompanied by increased interest in suicide among the general public. *The Wall Street Journal* reported a significant spike in calls to suicide hotlines following the suicide of a celebrity (Korte 2018). The common view is that the public feel an 'investment' in celebrities and need to reach out emotionally when a well-publicised suicide saturates the media.

---

[1] Thousands of German civilians killed themselves in 1945 in despair at the invading Russian army (Goesche 2009; Hubert 2019).

[2] There were subsequent official enquiries of a similar kind, especially of the Don Dale juvenile facility in the Northern Territory, and into drug rehabilitation facilities in regional New South Wales, both held in 2017.

(Historian David Frith published *Silence of the Heart: Cricket Suicides* in 2001, a worthy text in this context.)

There is a category in which visible signs are evident. Wekstein called this *focal suicide*—the kind where the person attacks part of their body as the source of their pain. Mutilation is the manifestation, whether of genital organs or of limbs. It is said to be self-harm without the intent of cessation, perhaps falling into the genre Wekstein called 'suicide gestures'. It can involve cutting, burning, bruising, even amputation. Australian psychiatrist Ernest Hunter has an interesting comment on cutting: he suggested to us that at times some youth cut themselves to see and feel life-affirming warm blood, a test by the 'cutter' that they are very much alive. If that is the case, what we may have here is 'self-prevention'.

A few scholars (Wekstein 1997; Long 1959) posited *accidental suicide*, some-times as *automatisation suicide*, that is, where a relatively unmotivated person takes barbiturates but feels that the drug isn't working and takes more and more to alleviate symptoms, often 'assisted' by alcohol. The person is often hypnogogic, that is, in an hallucinatory state and ingests more until death ensues. This may well be a form of suicide, but prevention, as is often the case, would seemingly lie with a close live-in partner or carer.

In a curious sense, the *neglect suicide* is the flipside of the *accidental* category: the suicider sometimes takes too little rather than too much. Hence, the diabetic who fails to measure blood glucose levels and forgets to take the essential medicating tablets or insulin doses. At the other end, the cardiac patient studiously disobeys dietary regimens and indulges outrageously, knowing deep down that this is inherently self-destructive.

One can write off such cases as mere stupidity or cussedness, but these scholars are certain that there is a strong element of self-cessation involved. They suggest that this is an overlap with a similar category they call *sub-intentional suicide*, those who truly live on the edge, who take inordinate risks by running red lights or taking boats to sea when all weather warnings say they shouldn't. Youth who train-surf may be in that category, although it can be difficult to separate normal youth risk-taking behaviour from sub-intentional acts. Karl Menninger (1893–1990), a major American researcher in this field, had an insightful term for this phenomenon: he called it *indirect suicide*. Clearly, there can be no prevention or intervention in this category.

It is difficult to locate what can be called *abstaining suicide*. It is prevalent among those who suffer eating disorders, particularly anorexia nervosa (AN), where one in three to one in five take their lives (Ashfield et al. 2015; Latzer and Hochdorf 2005). Are they dying to be thin, or is the pursuit of a skeletal appearance an intentional or a sub-intentional desire to cease? There are programs to treat the disorder, but not, it seems, for what lies beneath it. The psychiatric opinions we have sought suggest that there is often an oscillation between the motives of thinness and that of cessation.

(Eating disorders are a misunderstood and under-researched field, including recent suggestions that link obesity with high rates of suicide.)

Honour suicide is a feature of some societies. It is treated as an acceptable way out of a shameful or wrongful act, a righting of an aberration. It is a facet of the culture, not deviant or abnormal in any way. Traditionally, Japanese *samurai* warriors committed *seppuku* after a military defeat. A once common term in the civilian domain was *hari-kiri*. *Sacrificial suicide* was also to be found in Japanese military culture—the *kamikaze* pilots who flew their planes into the decks of enemy warships with the specific aim of killing foes rather than selves. Perhaps related, perhaps not, *political suicide* is usually a protest against a regime or an ideology, certainly what Barbagli calls an *against* form of suicide. Both Buddhism and Hinduism have long traditions of sacrificial-protest suicide, often by self-immolation. Another form of sacrifice was Hindu widows who elected to die on a husband's funeral pyre, a now somewhat obsolete ritual suicide called *sati* or *suttee*. In recent times, the world was aghast when Buddhist priests in Vietnam, especially under the reign of the Catholic president Ngo Dinh Diem in the 1950s and 1960s, set themselves alight in front of the world's cameras. (In Chap. 7, we discuss the political nature of some Australian Aboriginal suicides.)

A case can be made for a behaviour called *failure suicide*. The suddenly bankrupted businessman comes to mind, as does the investment broker who loses his clients' money. The drought-stricken farmer may well fall into this category. There are many reports of student-age suicides in fiercely competitive societies like Japan where it would seem that not topping the class or getting into a particular profession is a shaming thing.

The rational variety can be seen in an emerging category, the *pensioner suicide*. In the 1970s, the American psychologist Daniel Levinson studied adult male development (or ageing) in the USA (Levinson 1978). The essence of his *The Seasons of a Man's Life* was that we misconstrue the seasons. It is not simply infancy, adolescence, adulthood, middle age and old age. Every decade or so, he suggested, has its own features and attractions, and at the end of each such period one needs to sit down and contemplate what the next segment of life holds. By tailoring one's hopes, expectations, skills and limitations, one can renew life rather than suffer constant loss of physical and mental strength.

Data from the Australian National Coronial Information System (NCIS), which we have cited, verified 26,779 suicides between 1 January 2001 and 31 December 2013. Of those, 1177 were students (4.4%), while 3107 or close on 12% were described as pensioners or retirees. That is both surprising and disconcerting given the prominence of youth suicide all these years.

In our view, the *pensioner suicide* is one who has lost values that are the essence of their existence. In 1936, the renowned American political scientist Harold Lasswell (1902–1978) wrote his famous book *Politics: Who Gets What, When and How*. His view was that man, at least Western man, pursues five main values in life: income, deference, status, skills and safety (and those who achieve the most of such values become the elite). Income is clear enough. Deference is a hierarchical thing, as with the Pope at the head of a steep Roman Catholic pyramid, for example. Deference is often titular rather than power-based. Status is more to do with rank in relation to others. Skills are vital: they can be occupational, technical, professional, artistic, linguistic, oratorical, communicatory and military. Safety usually means freedom from war, invasion, civil strife, drought, floods and other natural disasters like earthquakes and tsunamis.

The pensioner, usually signed off at 55–65, loses not the values as such but their ability to use those values to a dedicated end. Here influential teachers stop teaching, the audience no longer there. Some countries, certainly Australia, no longer have compulsory retirement ages in the public and private sectors (and it would make for a good piece of research to examine suicide rate changes as between the compulsory retirement era and the non.) Men's sheds, sometimes called community sheds and open to both genders, are an Australian invention that intends to give retirees and older people a chance for greater social interaction and engagement in sensible projects.

But even so, the *pensioner suicide* category is obviously increasing among people who are still able-bodied and, if looked at intelligently, mentally and spiritually able to contribute to society.

The advent of radical Islamic *jihadism* brought about the common usage of human triggers to detonate bombs aimed at killing the infidel enemy. *Suicide bombers* are a form of mechanised weaponry designed to kill others, and the word suicide in the label is a misnomer. While this form of violent technology may have originated in Tsarist Russia, it became notorious in the much more recent revolutionary Islamic uprisings. ISIS and related organisations insist that the suicides are martyrs, but they fail to see, or don't wish to see, that martyrs are normally those who suffer, not those who inflict suffering. Suicide bombers are better named homicide bombers since the primary aim is not self-cessation as such but the death or maiming of others. With reluctance, we include this as a category because it does involve the wilful self-destruction of the bomber. There is an element of *cult suicide* here, a conscious or brain-washed willingness to die for a 'greater cause'.

Mass suicide is familiar to us from Roman history and the mass suicide of 960 Jewish zealots at Masada (in today's Israel) who preferred to die by their own hands rather than be enslaved or converted religiously by the Romans. This was a politico-religious decision in the face of what was seen as an impossible choice. A similar-looking mass suicide occurred in recent times; one that is better described as *cult suicide*. Roughly, the same number of people, 918, were induced to drink a cyanide-laced punch—and were forced at gunpoint to do so—in a mass murder-suicide at Jonestown in Guyana in November 1978.[3] The 'reverend' Jim Jones called it a 'revolutionary' action (by a strongly socialist group that once did some good work among the poor). This occurred among a draconian and at times paranoid cult, some of whose members

---

[3] See Guinn (2017).

had committed several murders, including that of a visiting American Congressman. It was a rehearsed ceremony in which coercion was the overwhelming factor. Many tried to resist; and at least one-third of the dead were children. This was hardly a Masada complex, but complexity of another kind.

The next category can be seen as the antithesis of *indirect suicide*, namely, what Shneidman (1998) called **logical suicide** and Wekstein termed **surcease suicide** or **rational suicide**. Here, a person concludes that their situation is irremediable, and with intellectual clarity concludes that the best way to end the pain is by death. (Euthanasia is, for the most part, just that: the ending of unendurable pain.) This is, of course, what Jean Améry was writing about, as we noted in Chap. 1. In Chap. 3, we discussed rational suicide in the works of philosophers Kant and Spinoza.

Psychotic suicide is typically found in those who suffer schizophrenic ideation: they don't intend dying but try rather to extirpate or exorcise their psychotic malignancy. Here, we are in the hands of the medical carer of the patient, not in the strategies of the prevention agencies.

A University of New South Wales study recently examined the records of some 36,000 persons who are autistic. Those afflicted are dying at twice the rate of the general population, mostly from injury or poisoning, the outcome of accident or suicide (*Sydney Morning Herald*, 27 February 2019). Earlier research indicated the difficulties involved in detecting suicidal intentions in those with an autistic disorder (Richa et al. 2014).

Defiant suicide is discussed in Chap. 7: Jews who took their lives before the Nazis could kill them; Armenian women who drowned themselves rather than submit to lives of sexual tyranny.

Chronic suicide is to be found among those who, at some level, wittingly extinguish themselves over time by alcohol or other substances. Hunter (1993) has analysed Aboriginal group drinking in the Kimberley region of Western Australia. He has found ritual, camaraderie and mutual reinforcement in these seemingly mindless exercises in obliteration. But obliteration of some kind it certainly is. We speculate that this phenomenon is akin to what we have called **grieving suicide** in many Aboriginal communities, the behaviour we discuss here, briefly, and in Chap. 7.

Aboriginal societies vary in their historical experiences, but a common enough feature is loss, lost connections to land, language, rites, rituals, children, parents and kin. They experience weekly losses by early deaths, often non-natural deaths. In the huge gap between their life expectancy and that of the White mainstream, there is an almost permanent cycle of grief and grieving, now often unabated with the loss of traditional mourning rituals and ceremonies. They also suffer what can be called political grief, with incessant setbacks on achieving political voices, social change, erosion of civil and human rights and so on.

This results in what Colin Tatz called **lost suicides** following a meeting with New Zealand psychiatrist Dr. Erahana Ryan. She described Māori youth as suffering 'stress of loss of who they are', 'the emptiness of blighted, warped, eviscerated urban Māori life'. There is 'a hole in their lives' and they don't know what it is (Tatz 2005: 87). Carey and McPhee (2018) concluded that Aboriginal suicide is due to **despair**, not depression.

Related to this category is *appealing suicide*, deriving from the work of anthropologist Emanuel Marx. Here, a person is at the end of their tether and feels unable to achieve any social aims unaided by others. It is partly a cry for help, said Marx and 'partly an attempt to shift some of their obligations towards their dependants on to others'. The person who cannot make that public appeal for help, nor persuade their family to share personal and social responsibilities, engages in violence towards others and finally to self as a desperate means to regain the support of family or kin.

Authenticity suicide or *validation suicide* may be one and the same thing. Both derive from the works of two notable writers, the American poet Sylivia Plath (1932–1963) and the Austrian writer Jean Améry (1912–1978). Plath was a perfectionist, dedicated to her 'project' of authenticity. (The important Alvarez book (1974) arose from his friendship with the poet.) She did try suicide and was saved. But she lived on a precipice of death and some literary critics believe she pushed that boundary to its logical end. She wanted to know what death actually *was*—not just engines chuffing up Jews—and we assume she found out.

These six lines of Plath's are taken from the opening of the Alvarez book:

Dying
Is an art, like everything else.
I do it exceptionally well.
I do it so it feels like hell.
I do it so it feels real.
I guess you could say I have a call.

Améry viewed suicide as entrance to another state of being and it isn't too far-fetched to conjecture that he wanted to authenticate his vision by finding another state, another place.

It is perhaps not a surprise that two other celebrated Holocaust survivor writers took their lives: the Italian chemist Primo Levi who once said that he didn't know he was alive enough to kill himself, did just that. He either 'threw himself down a staircase' or 'he tumbled over a railing' in 1987, producing the same reactions as we saw in the 9/11 'jumping' versus 'falling' case. The other case is that of the Romanian Paul Antschell, better known as the poet Paul Celan, who drowned himself in 1970. For us, his 48-line 'Todesfuge' ('Death Fugue') is the shortest, most seering summation ever on the Holocaust (Felstiner 1995). Some critics have asked whether the Améry–Levi–Celan deaths were perhaps delayed homicides—the inference that they believed they should have died by Nazi murder rather than survived?

Psychiatry may have a name for this form of cessation, but it isn't hard to see something of that notion in the self-deaths of creative artists who have either sought to push the very edges of corporeal existence or who have died because they couldn't find a way of truly validating their talents and their livingness.

Occupational suicide is where there is a high incidence of self-death in professions that carry undue stress, such as medicine and the military. The rate among doctors in America is reported as twice that of the general population. Anaesthetists and psychiatrists are the specialists with the highest risk (Kreimer 2018). We address this category of suicide in some detail in Chap. 12 on the professionals.

Assisted suicide is a significant category and now a rigidly defined legal one. It involves elements and aspects of *fatalistic*, *existential*, *despairing* and *anomic suicide*. We note here that it involves a high degree of *rational suicide* and one that appears to exclude illness of the mind. The 2017 *Assisted-Dying* statute of the Australian state of Victoria insists that the requester of such a death must have rational decision-making capacity. We have a separate chapter on this phenomenon, but note here that it involves a high degree of *rational suicide* and one that appears to exclude illness of the mind.

There may well be yet another category: *cyber* or *Internet suicide*. We witness a rising incidence of youth who escape Internet bullying not by turning off their addictive computers but by turning off their lives. And then, we have the younger Twitter–Facebook–Instagram generation that has begun to discover that friendships and relationships in cyberspace are not real relationships, that their visual world is but a small screen of nothingness: the buzzes, the highs, the sex and the food are not real. Many young persons find solace in the screens, and there are those who don't.

Jesse Bering has a startling title to a chapter in his book, *Suicidal* (2018): 'To Log Off This Mortal Coil' (borrowing from Hamlet's 'shuffling off' life's burden).

Suicide by murder, often called *suicide-by-cop* in popular parlance, is actually a form of victim-provoked homicide. The person considers suicide as a non-virile or even a cowardly act and so selects and then provokes a superior adversary, often a police officer, to bring about their demise. A good deal of concern has been raised in Australia about the training given, or not given, to police on how to handle what are usually considered mentally ill persons who appear to be seeking this kind of violent response.[4]

Copycat or cluster suicides have been reported by the U.S. Centres for Disease Control. The report known as *Suicide Contagion and the Reporting of Suicide: Recommendations from a National Workshop* discussed the need to reduce 'the possibility' of media-related suicide contagion, described as 'a process by which exposure to the suicide or suicidal behaviour of one or more persons influences others to

---

[4]In the past 20 years, NSW Police have shot dead 35 persons, half of them suffering diagnosed mental illness.

commit or attempt suicide. 'Contagion', which is apparently most evident among adolescents, results in suicide 'clusters'.

Copycat suicide is also referred to as 'the Werther effect', named after Goethe's 1774 story called 'The Sorrows of Young Werther'. The concept rests on the notion that when someone reads of a suicide, usually of a young person, it sets off a train of suicides in emulation. So strong is the belief in this effect that some countries, including New Zealand, prohibit the publication of the method of a suicide. (Mindframe in Australia has the same intent but their objectives are advisory, not mandatory.) Media may publish the fact of a suicide, but not the manner of—lest someone gets ideas. In this day and age of social media and instant information, there is something bizarre about 'protecting' youth from methods of surcease.

Text suicide, said Wekstein, is indeed a vague classification, but it may have some value in the approach to a likely suicide. It rests on what responses a person gives to what are psychological tests for risks of suicide. Depressive responses may be a marker for suicidal thoughts.

Lastly, the *unknown suicides*. The NCIS report on suicide in Australia for the years 2001–2013 listed 2974 or 11% as 'unlikely to be known'.

Suicide can hardly be classified as a *genus* in the way that, for example, biological plants can be classified into broad genera, with up to dozens or hundreds of species or sub-species. But the classifications suggested here offer a rough template of differently based, differently driven acts of cessation. It proposes a typology by which to better target prevention and intervention strategies, and drive what we all seem to be striving for, namely, *understanding* of the suicide phenomenon.

6.2 Twenty Methods

'How did he do it?', 'what did she do?'. Morbid curiosity leads to the almost reflexive questions at news of a suicide. As perverse as it may well be, humans are fascinated by the means people use to kill themselves.

At times, but hardly always, the methods people select for death are linked to prevention possibilities. Removing access to lethal means underpins much of suicide prevention strategy: if, somehow, we can deny the method, we can preserve a life. The Gap is an ocean cliff in Sydney's well-to-do Watson's Bay area, beautiful in vista but infamous for suicide. For years, there were campaigns to fence the area, seemingly in the belief that without this venue would-be suicides would be deterred.[5]

---

[5]The late Don Ritchie is said to have saved 160 lives by asking those about to jump from The Gap if there was anything he could do to help. But our point is that an intercession is not a guarantee that the parasuicide won't find another means or another venue, at another time.

There is an illogic at work: there is always another cliff and there are no shortages of heights in Sydney or any other city.

Openness about method has further implications. Public reporting on suicide is *allegedly* linked to the 'Werther Effect', mentioned above. In Australia and elsewhere, media guidelines instruct journalists not to report on method (and even location), believing the information will 'inspire' others to suicide. Thus, the first rule of suicide prevention is not to talk about suicide.

Following the suicide of internationally popular musician Kurt Cobain (of famed rock band Nirvana) in 1994, a decrease in suicide deaths in his Seattle region was reported; this was attributed, in part, to how he killed himself (Jobes et al. 1996). Cobain used a shotgun, a 'method of choice, which would seem especially violent, even to a person at risk' wrote Jobes et al. (1996) in their study on the impact of this high-profile death. This wasn't a gentle passing; it was a violent act that shocked music fans and the general public. An Australian study by Martin and Koo (1999) also found no increase in suicide in the 30 days of intense media coverage following his death.

The literature on preventing suicide method is mixed and contentious (see Chap. 8). The million individuals who do suicide each year find a method and a means. The millions more who attempt suicide add to the complexity. The cliché of a 'cry for help' is real—that is, the persons who 'attempt' suicide but use methods classified as 'less lethal'. Estimates vary on how many are 'attempts' and how many (to use that rather disconcerting term) 'complete'; yet for every completed suicide, there are anywhere up to nine people who are 'attempters'. (Some scholars claim a greater number than nine.)

Preventionists focus on method and its reporting, as if denying the public information on 'how' and 'where' will reduce the 'why'. We have serious questions to ask about whether concentration on means is a result of not understanding motive.

Suicide methods differ remarkably. Within countries, regions, age groups, cultures, religions and gender, disparities bring to the fore how problematic (and unachievable in many instances) 'prevention' is. As discussed at the start of this chapter, there is no single strategy to prevent cancer, and there is no single avenue to suicide prevention. Nor is there much to learn from the statistical analyses of suicide methods in six countries, to be found at the end of this chapter.

If preventing suicide is the desired outcome, is there consensus on which types of suicide are being prevented, or how are they being prevented? Does preventing suicide by jumping from The Gap mean that the person won't end life by another means? Or is it a one-size-fits-all approach that all suicides, regardless of method and means, are being prevented? And can suicide, irrespective of method, be addressed using standardised or uniform preventions?

We have identified at least 20 known methods of suicide:

1.   hanging (hyoid bone breaking);

2.   asphyxiation/suffocation/ligatures (popularly called hanging);

3.   firearms;

4.   jumping;

5.   drowning;

6.   poisoning: domestic toxins/pesticides;

7.   transport (vehicle accident, trains, trucks, buses, cars, aircraft);

8.   overdosing (prescription or illegal drugs/injection (drug, insulin, etc.));

9.   gassing (gas ovens, carbon monoxide);

10. bleeding: wrist- or throat-cutting;

11. abstaining (starvation, dehydration, medications);

12. 'by cop'/provocation;

13. immolation;

14. arson (structured fire);

15. electrocution;

16. freezing;

17. impalement: on sword, sharp fence;

18. exposure (to the elements);

19. explosives/terrorist bombing; and

20. other/ritual (*sati* in India, *seppuku* in Japan; volcano, animal attack (bear dens in zoos), snake enclosures, joining a dangerous enterprise like ISIS).

The World Health Organization provides a comprehensive analysis of suicide method by country (Ajdacic-Gross et al. 2008). Firearms are now the leading means of suicide in the USA, pesticides are the dominant method in Asia, while emerging ways, such as charcoal-burning suicide, is now reported in that continent. The study differentiated suicide into much broader categories than we list. The authors cautioned that data on certain methods (hanging and firearms) are more accurately reported than poisoning or drowning, and many countries have 'incomplete data'.

We have a plethora of research studies on suicide methods. Wading through the literature confirms that method is often enough linked to outcome. Firearms and hanging are the most lethal forms, poisoning and stabbing are in the 'less effective' category. Suicide methods differ between (and within) nations: America is infamous for high rates of firearm use in suicides (and homicides) but guns are infrequent in

Asia where restrictions on weapons operate. Pesticides are commonly used in Asia, while hanging is more prevalent in Europe and Australia (Park et al. 2014).

For reader convenience, we have placed below the statistical treatment of method variations between six countries. They warrant browsing in order to get a grasp of what is happening in three continents.

6.3   Variations in Suicide Methods

South Korea has high rates of suicide and distinctive means. It has the highest suicide rate among OECD[6] countries, and suicide is in the top five causes of death. An estimated 40 persons kill themselves every day. Rates are high among the elderly: they are a large proportion of the population, nearly half of whom live in poverty. Suicide is also the leading cause of death for teenagers, with almost 8% saying they considered suicide, according to *Business Insider* (Park et al. 2014). The Summary Result of the 2016 South Korean Social Survey listed 'economic hardships' as the main reason for the impulse.

An insightful South Korean analysis, '*Difference in suicide methods used between suicide attempters and suicide completers*' (Lim et al. 2014), found a variation in method between the attempters and those who died. Poisoning was the most frequent by parasuicides, hanging commonest among suiciders. Based on their classification of lethality, the authors established that some 70% of attempters used a non-lethal method, while almost all suiciders used methods considered lethal. The choice of method correlates with completions.

Other studies reached similar conclusions. Spicer and Miller (2000) found nine out of ten suicide attempts were non-fatal, with males more likely to select a lethal method (firearms, drowning or hanging/suffocation) than females, who chose less lethal methods (poisoning, cutting) (Spicer and Miller 2000).

Recent declines in South Korea's suicide rate were attributed to legislation prohibiting the sale of paraquat, a highly toxic weed killer, excruciatingly painful, slow and irreversible. *Business Insider* (2018) stated the use of paraquat and other pesticides accounted for a fifth of all South Korean suicides between 2006 and 2010. The reduction in death by pesticide poisoning—more significantly in rural areas, among men and the elderly—has been attributed to the banning of pesticides. Access barriers have reduced deaths, at least in the short term. In Japan, the introduction of blue light-emitting-diode (LED) lamps on railway platforms and crossings is apparently reducing suicides at these locations, but we do not know if these people suicided elsewhere or later.

---

[6]Organisation for Economic Co-operation and Development.

   But, as Park et al. (2014) explained, the reduction in poisoning in South Korea has been offset by 'increased use of hanging', a method much more difficult to regulate.

   The major source of UK data is the *National Confidential Inquiry into Suicide and Homicide by People with Mental Illness* (NCISH).[7] We question why there isn't or wasn't an enquiry into suicide by people *without* a mental illness. The enquiry does not evaluate social and existential factors, or such indicators as social isolation, unemployment, living alone, having a co-morbid condition, alcohol and drug misuse.

   Starting with England, the 2017 NCISH report showed that between 2005 and 2015, the number of deaths in the general population registered as suicide or 'undetermined' was 49,545, an average of 4504 annually. As to methods:

- hanging and strangulation were the most common, 23,970 or 48%;

- self-poisoning (including overdoses) accounted for 9827 deaths or 20%;

- jumping and multiple injuries (including jumping from a height or suicide by train) resulted in 5336 deaths or 11%;

- drowning was categorised as a 'less frequent' method, 2193, 4%;

- gas inhalation led to 1914 deaths, 4%;

- cutting and stabbing, 1384 dead, 3%; and

- firearms, 971 suicides, 2%.

Hanging and jumping (multiple injuries) increased, while suicides by self-poisoning decreased. What were deemed 'less common methods', such as drowning and firearms, decreased. Between 2005 and 2010, suicide by gas inhalation fell, 'reflecting a fall in car exhaust asphyxiation'; however, this figure increased 'after this time with an increase in other gases, for example, helium'.

   For English 'patients' (that is, people who have been in contact with mental health services in the 12 months prior to death), hanging, self-poisoning and jumping/multiple injuries were the most common methods. Death by opiates (self-poisoning) accounted for 26% of deaths, by anti-psychotic drugs (11%), tricyclic antidepressants (10%) and SSRI/SNRIs antidepressants (9%). Suicide using the same drugs used to treat depression and psychosis warrants a separate analysis. If approximately 30% of patients in England are taking their lives using the medication supposedly designed to treat their mental illnesses, then the efficacy of the medication and the value of prescribing it is surely questionable. Such medical regimens may well contribute to suicide attempts.

---

[7] *The National Confidential Inquiry into Suicide and Homicide by People with Mental Illness.* Annual Report: England, Northern Ireland, Scotland and Wales. October 2017. University of Manchester.

Northern Ireland experienced an increase in the number and rate of suicides between 2005 and 2015. In that time, the NCISH reported 2903 deaths as suicide or 'undetermined', an average of 264 per year:

- hanging and strangulation accounted for 56% (higher than England);
- self-poisoning 27% (higher than England);
- so too drowning (8%);
- gas inhalation was lower (2%); and
- jumping/multiple injuries, and cutting and stabbing, just 1%.

Suicides by hanging and self-poisoning had increased since 2006 and 2008, respectively, with a decrease in deaths by gas inhalation. The most common methods were hanging, poisoning and drowning, accounting for 90% of suicides. Suicides by opiates increased by 83% between 2005 and 2014.

Scotland is divergent. NCISH was notified of 8662 deaths as suicide or 'undetermined' between 2005 and 2015, an average of 787 per year:

- hanging and strangulation were 40%;
- self-poisoning 32% (considerably higher than England);
- jumping/multiple injuries were 10%;
- drownings were almost double England's rate at 7%;
- gas inhalation 3%;
- cutting and stabbing 2%; and
- firearms 1%.

NCISH reported that suicides by hanging increased between 2005 and 2015, while they noted changes in coding roles altered the self-poisoning data. The high rate of drownings by suicide actually reflected a decrease of 69% between 2005 and 2015. For patients in Scotland, the rate of suicide by self-poisoning was 36%; the same rate for hanging. A much higher rate of suicide by opiates was found in Scotland than England—in the former 40% suicided by opiates. Suicide by antidepressants 15% and anti-psychotics 11% again showed a very high rate using medication prescribed to treat mental illness.

Finally, Wales, where 3493 deaths by suicide or 'undetermined' conclusion, or an average of 318 per year, were reported between 2005 and 2015:

- hanging and strangulation, 55%;
- self-poisoning, 18%;

- jumping/multiple injuries, 7%;

- drowning, 5%;

- gas inhalation, 4%;

- cutting and stabbing, 3%; and

- firearms, just 2%.

Suicide by hanging increased over the period while drownings decreased. Patients in Wales who suicided did so most commonly by hanging 48%, self-poisoning 23% and jumping/multiple injuries 10%. Opiates, anti-psychotics and SSRI/SNRI antide-pressants were reportedly used in 51% of patient suicides.

The extent to which prevention strategies are effective is dubious given the British variations. Why would people hang themselves more often in England than North-ern Ireland? Why were Scottish rates so much higher for drownings than in their neighbouring country? And why did so many people take their lives using medica-tions designed to treat mental illness? Could it be that the link between suicide and mental illness was, in part, a factor of the medication and its misuse? If prevention of access to method reduces suicide, then logically not prescribing anti-psychotics and antidepressants could reduce the suicide rate substantially?

The USA is noted for its gun culture, so there is no surprise that firearms are the most common method, accounting for over 50% of all deaths. [Of interest is that firearms were low down the list in early twentieth-century American suicides: 24% in 1901–1905 and a jump to 35% in 1926–1930; poisonings went down from 34 to 16% in those periods, suggesting no correlation between access and method (Dublin and Bunzel 1933: 58).] Data sets differed from the comprehensive UK statistics cited above, making direct comparisons difficult. But looking across the various reports across the decade 2000–2010, we gather that suffocation/hanging was the method in about 22% of suicides, and poisoning at just over 17%, falls (which we believe includes jumping) were 2.1%. Drowning was a method in just 1.1%, fire 0.5% and motor vehicle 0.3%.

In our list of 20 suicide methods, we have not included euthanasia or suicide bombers or *kamikaze*-like acts. Yet there is a form of suicide that is not dissim-ilar, what is termed 'death-by-cop' or 'involuntary participation by others'. This is described as an act by individuals who wish to die but not by their own hand. It involves provocation, sometimes using an empty or fake weapon, to provoke an armed police officer to kill them; or else committing acts of murder with the intent of being killed by police. Suicide.org, a US-based website,[8] suggested this form of suicide is not uncommon. Citing a study published in the Annals of Emergency Medicine, using data from the Los Angeles County Sheriff's Department, researchers found that '11% of officer-involved shootings were suicide-by-cop incidents' (between 1987

---

[8]http://www.suicide.org/suicide-by-cop.html.

through 1997). Of these, 98% were male, about 50% carried weapons that were loaded, while 17% brandished a toy or replica gun.

In 2015, the office of Oakland County Medical Examiner (USA) ruled that a 22-year-old woman, Rebecca Hardy, had committed suicide when she climbed a fence and was mauled to death by two dangerous dogs. Newspaper reports quote the medical examiner, Dr. Ljubisa Dragovic: 'She climbed the fence and jumped in and basically subjected herself to the attacks, which constitutes a purposeful act'. Hardy 'had gotten into an argument at her home, left barefooted and walked about a mile to where she knew the aggressive dogs would be confined' local media reported.[9]

Acknowledging that the Internet can be an unreliable source of facts, there are several reports of deaths by people entering into zoo enclosures, such as the naked man who climbed into a lion's enclosure at a Chilean zoo, reportedly spouting apocalyptic chants.

Like everything else, statistics need a context. In the 1920s and 1930s, households tended to have gas stoves and gas heaters, hence an available method of ending life. Homes had fly-catcher strips hanging from ceilings, a ready source of arsenic when rinsed in water. Increased car ownership led to accessible carbon monoxide. Removing or banning one avenue inevitably leads to the use of another method. Social invention and social change bring about new and differing technologies.

Common sense dictates that when we are confronted by different kinds, different groupings, different grades or classes of a phenomenon like suicide, we would construct different and appropriate responses. Logic also comes to mind in the training of those who see their task as preventing suicide. Yet we seem not to educate doctors and nurses in any depth. Nor do we educate lawyers and lawyers who become coroners about suicide in history, suicide in the present, suicide in any sociological or anthropological senses. This is indeed a strange quirk in a field that now commands so much government and media attention, so many man-hours and dollars in the world of preventions. As a fact, the suicide rates go up.

References

Ajdacic-Gross, V., Weiss, M. G. Ring, M., Hepp, U., Bopp, M., Gutzwiller, F., et al. (2008), Methods of suicide: International suicide patterns derived from the WHO mortality database. *Bulletin of the World Health Organization, 86*(9), 726–732. http://www.who.int/bulletin/volumes/86/9/0042-9686_86_07-043489-table-T1.html.
Alvarez, A. (1974). *The savage God: A study of suicide*. London: Penguin Books.
Améry, J. (1999). *On suicide: A discourse on voluntary death*. Bloomington, IN: Indiana University Press.

[9]http://www.khq.com/story/30720227/death-of-michigan-woman-attacked-by-two-dogs-deemed-a-suicide.

Ashfield, J., Smith, A., & Bain, L. (2015, July). *Facts about suicide*. Australian Institute of Male Health and Studies.

Baechler, J. (1975). *Suicides*. New York: Basic Books.

Barbagli, M. (2015). *Farewell to the world: A history of suicide*. New Jersey: Wiley.

Bering, J. (2018). *Suicidal: Why we kill ourselves*. Chicago: Chicago University Press.

Business Insider (2018). Axel Springer SE.

Camus, A. (1955). *The myth of Sisyphus*. London: Hamish Hamilton.

Carey, T., & McPhee, R. (2018, December 14). It's despair not depression that's responsible for Indigenous suicide. *The Conversation*.

Douglas, J. (1967). *The social meanings of suicide*. Princeton, NJ: Princeton University Press.

Dublin, L., & Bunzel, B. (1933). *To be or not to be: A study in suicide*. New York: Harrison Smith and Robert Haas.

Durkheim, É. [1897] (2013). *Suicide: A study in sociology*. New York: The Free Press.

Felstiner, J. (1995). *Paul Celan: Poet, Survivor, Jew*. New Haven, CO: Yale University Press.

Frith, D. (2001). *Silence of the heart: Cricket suicides*. London: Mainstream Publishing.

Goesche, C. (2009). *Suicide in Nazi Germany*. Oxford: Oxford University Press.

Guinn, J. (2017). *The road to Jonestown: Jim Jones and peoples temple*. New York: Simon & Schuster.

https://doi.org/10.1111/j.1943-278X.1996.tb00611.x.

Hubert, F. (2019). *Promise me you will shoot yourself: The mass death of German civilians in 1945*. Melbourne: Text Publishing.

Hunter, E. (1993). *Aboriginal health and history: Power and prejudice in remote Australia*. Cambridge: Cambridge University Press.

International Journal of Mental Health Systems, 8:22. (2014). https://doi.org/10.1186/1752-4458-8-22.

Jobes, D. A., Berman, I. L., O'Carroll, P. W., Eastgard, S., & Knickmeyer, S. (1996). The Kurt Cobain suicide crisis: Perspectives from research, public health, and the news media. https://doi.org/10.1111/j.1943-278X.1996.tb00611.x.

Kreimer, S. (2018). https://www.physicianleaders.org/news/-preventing-physician-suicide-recognizing-symptoms-improving-support-i.

Korte, L. (2018, June 10). After celebrity deaths, suicide hotline calls jump 25%. *Wall Street Journal*.

Lasswell, H. (1936). *Politics: Who gets what, when and how*. London: McGraw-Hill Company.

Latzer, Y., & Hochdorf, Z. (2005). Dying to be thin: Attachment to death in anorexia nervosa. *The Scientific World Journal, 5,* 820–827.

Levinson, D. (1978). *The seasons of a man's life*. New York: Ballantine Books.

Lim, M., Lee, U., & Par, J.-I. (2014). Difference in suicide methods used between suicide attempters and suicide completers. *International Journal of Mental Health Systems, 20148,* 54. https://doi.org/10.1186/1752-4458-8-54.

Long, R. (1959, April). Barbiturates, automatization and suicide. *Insurance Council Journal,* 299–307.

Martin, G., & Koo, L. (1999). Celebrity suicide: Did the death of Kurt Cobain influence young suicides in Australia? *Archives of Suicide Research,* 197–198, 1997.

Miller, D., & Miller, L. T. (1992). Women and children in the Armenian genocide. In R. Hovanissian (Ed.), *The Armenian genocide: History, politics, ethics*. New York: St. Martin's Press.

Miller, D., & Miller, L. T. (1999). *Survivors: An oral history of the Armenian Genocide*. Berkeley: University of California.

Mukherjee, S. (2010). *The emperor of all maladies: A biography of cancer*. New York: Simon & Schuster.

Park, S., Ahn, M. H., Lee, A., & Hong, J. P. (2014). Associations between changes in the pattern of suicide methods and rates in Korea, the US, and Finland.

Richa, S., Fahed, M., Khoury, E., & Mishara, B. (2014). Suicide in autism spectrum disorders. *Archives of Suicide Research, 18,* 327–339. 2014 Copyright # International Academy for Sui-

cide Research ISSN: 1381-1118 print=1543-6136 online https://doi.org/10.1080/13811118.2013.
8248.

Shneidman, E. (1998). *The suicidal mind*. Oxford: Oxford University Press.

Simmel, G. (1908). The stranger. *Soziologie. Untersuchungen über die Formen der Vergesellschaftung* (pp. 509–512). Berlin: Duncker & Humblot.

Snyder, T. (2010, June). Suicide, slavery, and memory in North America. *Journal of American History*, 39–62.

Snyder, T. (2015). *The power to die: Slavery and suicide in British North America*. Chicago: Chicago University Press.

Spicer, R., & Miller, T. R. (2000, December). Suicide acts in 8 states: Incidence and case fatality rates by demographics and method. *American Journal of Public Health, 90*(12).

Tatz, C. (2001, 2005 revised). *Aboriginal suicide is different: A portrait of life and self-destruction*. Canberra: Aboriginal Studies Press.

Wekstein, L. (1979). *A handbook of suicidology: Principles, problems and practice*. New York: Brunnere/Mazel. 26–30.

Wekstein, L. (1997). *A handbook of suicidology: Principles, problems and practice*. New York: Brunner/Mazel.

Chapter 7
Differing Contexts

Death crises occur more often for American Indians at an earlier age and, furthermore, the deaths of their ancestors (which came close to genocide) remains a powerful tribal memory. American Indians are aware of their isolation from mainstream culture. They are both isolated geographically and suffer from racism... Suicide by the American Indian, for example, may be seen as seeking freedom in death.

—David Lester (1997)

To us, health is about much more than simply not being sick. It's about getting a balance between physical health, emotional, cultural, and spiritual health.

—Tamara Mackean [Dr. Mackean is a Waljen woman of the Goldfields region of Western Australia (WA). She holds a conjoint appointment as a senior research fellow at the George Institute for Global Health and the Southgate Institute for Health, Society and Equity at Flinders University of South Australia]

Abstract Suicide needs to be *understood* rather than deplored and shunned. Case studies of differing suicide patterns across geographies, histories, religions and cultures, particularly among Australia's Aboriginal people and North American Indians and Inuit; suicide during the Armenian and Jewish genocides in the twentieth century.

Keywords Ethnic minorities · Lost connections · Facing impossible choices

7.1 Connections

The fortunes of ethnic minorities have often been determined by geography and history. Their present is almost always a result of their distant and recent past, as with Armenians, Jews, and the Romani. So too the colonial experiences of the Australian Aboriginal people and the Indian and Inuit people of North America. They don't

© Springer Nature Switzerland AG 2019   79
C. Tatz and S. Tatz, *The Sealed Box of Suicide*,
https://doi.org/10.1007/978-3-030-28159-5_7

(or can't) discard or shuffle off the consequences of the genocidal events that have befallen them and their forefathers, legacies which include high rates of suicide. Their estates are pervaded by the after-effects to this day. The tribal memory always lingers, often looms. Grief is integral, umbilical perhaps, to suicide, and these First Nations people have a respect for, and veneration of, grief, rather than haste 'to move on' or 'to get over it'. Several of these factors make for different contexts of suicide, different from the mainstream milieu in which they live.

The relationship between genocide and suicide is neglected, possibly not seen, apart from a short but important article on the Arctic Inuit and Australian experiences that discusses *cultural* genocide as a factor in suicide (Leenaars et al. 1998). [The killing aspect and the serious physical harm to Australian Aborigines were of greater magnitude than that which beset the Inuit, and hence, Leenaars' emphasis on cultural genocide—the attempted killing of Inuit values and language.]

The link is clear when we look at the Armenian and Jewish genocides in the twentieth century. But we need to look further—at Herero, Damara and Nama women in German South-West Africa [Namibia] following the genocide and rape of those women by the German military between 1904 and 1906; at Congolese women who suffered Belgium's genocidal actions between 1885 and 1908; at the outcomes for Bosnian Muslim women who were forced into dedicated rape centres during the Wars of Yugoslav Succession between 1991 and 2001; at the round-up of Yazidi women and girls as slaves in Iraq in 2014; at the life and times of the hundreds of thousands of Rohingya women and children who fled Myanmar in 2017 and 2018; and at the violent treatment of Syrian girl brides as this is being written.

The connections lie in the aftermath of genocide that have been transmitted—or osmosed—through the generations, the shadows that permeate much of their lives and attitudes towards their corporeal existence.

7.2 Understanding or Explaining?

A number of ethnic communities in the Western world have cultural practices of suicide, but not all. In some cases suicide is rare; in others, it is rampant. Several communities have such an escalation of suicide rates that they have had to establish community rather than the Western biomedical models of intervention. This is where the admonitions of the American psychologist James Hillman (1926–2011) are pertinent. First, he contended that we must try to *understand* suicide rather than *explain* it; second, in our studies we should avoid 'moving sideways into comparisons' (Hillman 1997: 49). In our search for an explanation, we do look, however briefly, at a few similarities and differences between cases. Apart from the common factor of self-cessation among Australian Aborigines and North American Indians, the contextual portraits of their suicides are not only different from their mainstreams, but there are almost no diagnoses of illness of the mind. Either that or they are not seeking health care—unlikely given the attention to ethnic suicide for at least the last three decades. The research to date shows little, if any, connection between their suicides and mental disorders. One needs to heed the research of Hjelmeland and Knizek (2017): they found that the 'well-established truth' that 90% of [all] suicides are related to, or rather, caused by mental disorders, is 'weak', and hardly a 'truth'.

In his *Suicide and the Soul*, Hillman wrote: 'self-killing … means both a killing of community and involvement of community in the killing'. Just as Dr Jack Kevorkian's assisted suicide campaign in the USA opened up that issue, so Hillman's plea was that suicide should be judged 'by some community court', comprising legal, medical, aesthetic, religious and philosophical interests, as well as by family and friends. In that way, self-death can 'come out of the closet'. The act of suicide will, of course, remain individualistic, 'but judgment of the suicide as part of, or interior to, a community may help to liberate Western civilisation's "persecutory panic" when suicide, or the threat of it, arises'. Why, he asked, 'the fierce resistance in Western civilisation to opening the closed door', or as we call it, the sealed box?' (Hillman 1997: 200). We must, he concluded, get away from 'police action, lockups, criminalisation of helpers, dosages to dumbness' [a reference to the mind-dulling effects of antidepressant chemicals]. In 2018, Australia experienced its worst drought in recorded history. The number of stricken farmer suicides in dire circumstances began to 'open up' suicide in Hillman's collective and communal way—even if just a little. Some of the public and some of the media started to perceive such deaths differently—in a more comprehending and kindlier way.

In America and Australia, we progress very little in the way of comprehension, insisting as we do on explanation and on causality—inevitably 'mental health issues', on seeking out 'at-risk' factors, on prescribing more dosages of dumbness. Some inroads have been made into the sovereignty of biopower and of the individualisation and isolation of suicide—by native communities in Australia, North America, Canada, the Pacific Islands and New Zealand. The ethnic communities themselves—not the specialists' consulting rooms, the hospitals or Alvarez's 'isolation wards of science'—have become the locus and focus of suicide, especially that of youth. The 'community' has taken on the phenomenon and the problem it presents.[1] Jack Anovak, an Inuit elder, has said: 'It is our problem and we have to deal with it'; 'we are the experts on our stories' (Leenaars 1998: 343, 357).

---

[1] For example, a major segment of the second National Aboriginal and Torres Strait Islander Suicide Prevention Conference in Perth in 2018 was 'The Importance of Community Partnerships'.

7.3   The Prime Examples

The characteristics of all suicide cases that are as a result of a genocide allow us to distinguish between two categories of the action—those who, in the words of the Italian scholar Marzio Barbagli, do it *for* self and *for* others and those who do it as a form of revenge or challenge *against* others (Barbagli 2015). *For* and *against* have the inherent quality of intent, and intent always carries with it a degree of rationality, even if it is of the misguided kind.

Die Endlösung der Judenfrage—'the final solution to the Jewish question'—was the name the Nazis gave to their programme to eliminate both the physical being and the very concept of 'Jew'. The American historian Lawrence Langer defined what befell that victim group as 'facing choiceless choices'. Thus, while most people view suicide as resulting from 'disease of the mind', for those imperilled by grotesque circumstances, self-destruction was, and is indeed, the best way out, the effective 'ultimate refuge' (Kwiet 1984).

Apart from the Nazi invention of specific-purpose death factories, the Turkish nationalists set most of the precedents for the Holocaust that took place a quarter of a century later. They articulated a formal ideological, sociological, anthropological and linguistic presentation of a superior civilisation 'confronted' by an 'enemy within', with an allegedly ill-fitting, pernicious minority, a fifth column, and an 'abscess' in the midst of a burgeoning nationalistic state. They initiated Armenian deportations, population transfers and the confiscation and transfer of property; the round-up of men, the disarming of Armenian civilians and soldiers, the creation of slave labour camps; the desecration of churches and cemeteries; the taking and forced Turkification of children; the elementary gas chambers, the medical experiments, the drownings and burnings, the rape of women, the death marches—all of which led to the extirpation of 1.5 million Armenians, one half of that ethnic population then living in Turkey in the period 1915 to 1923. One major difference between the Armenian and Jewish cases was that Armenian children could be saved if they surrendered to fostering and Turkification, and in some instances, women could live if they submitted to the degradation of sexual chatteldom or prostitution.

The debasement of Armenian women was central to the Turkish elimination of Armenians and Armenianness. Rape, gang rape, 'gifts' of girls to officials, forced prostitution, defilement and the organised medical disfigurement of pretty girls were part of the plan to 'settle the Armenian question' once and for all (Dadrian 1986). Raymond Kévorkian, a noted historian of the Armenian genocide, commented on one Armenian response to the events (Kévorkian 2011: 407):

> Suicides were also quite frequent. If the main reason for this was simply despair, many of those who took their own lives were young women, who chose to throw themselves into the Euphrates rather than submit to rape. Mothers also frequently refused to submit to the will of their torturers, killing themselves and their children instead.

Two scholars of the Armenian genocide, Donald and Lorna Touryan Miller, have addressed specifically the matter of women and children during the Armenian onslaught (Miller and Touryan Miller 1992: 152–172). They noted the many references to suicide when interviewing survivors. Their conclusions are of particular interest, given that a few suicide scholars have attempted to frame differing categories of suicide, something essential if we are to make any progress in alleviating or mitigating the 'problem'. The Millers posit three acts: *altruistic suicide*, *despairing suicide* and, significant for this analysis of ethnic suicides, *defiant suicide*. Thus, grandmothers and mothers who sacrificed themselves by giving their food rations to children were performing acts of altruism in dying *for* others. Grandmothers staying behind so that children could walk away faster was another example of *for*.

The despairing ones were those who could walk on the death marches but chose to stay behind and die; and those who were physically exhausted and whose support structure had collapsed, chose to drown themselves.

This *defiant* category is significant: it fits Barbagli's dyad of both *for* and *against*. Armenian women took their lives rather than submit to the commonplace torture, sexual abuse and rape by their oppressors. Historically, the Armenian Apostolic Church regards suicide as a grievous sin, placing the suicide as beyond salvation and beyond burial by the church (except where mental illness is shown to be evident). These women defied both biological instinct and church doctrine. Yet on 24 April 2015, the hundredth anniversary of the onset of that genocide, the Apostolic Church sanctified *all* who died as martyrs—including those who suicided.

Most people made aware of such circumstances would understand what was involved. Many would acknowledge the actions of these women as honourable, perhaps admirable, certainly as comprehensible. There would be some appreciation of actions that are consonant with martyrdom. Many would argue that such behaviours were the result of coerced choices. These victim women exercised their wills, their rational wills, in appalling contexts. So what stops suicide scholars and helping practitioners from appreciating circumstances that are less dramatic, situations that are as hopeless (or seemingly as hopeless) as these? Does the compelling force of understanding self-death reside only in the perception of the beholder rather than in the one whose life is to end?

Suicide among Jews in the early Nazi period was also common (Kwiet 1984: 135–168). That was remarkable because traditional Judaism, as most religions, regards suicide as unacceptable. Among major religions, Judaism generally has fewer suicides. Yet suicides were common enough in crisis times, and Jews experienced endless crises: they were deemed responsible for the death of Jesus, and as the transmitters of the Black Plague; they were expelled from European societies like Spain, Portugal and England; held responsible for famines and for the deaths of Christian children at Passover time (the 'blood libel' by which Jews were alleged to have made unleavened bread out of their blood); they endured pogroms in Russia, Ukraine and Poland, and a third of them died in the Holocaust.

There are two exceptions to the Jewish decree of suicide as sinful. One is *Kiddush Hashem*, the taking of one's life in defence of God, that is, choosing martyrdom rather than forced apostasy (especially during the Crusades in the Middle Ages). The other, introduced by Rabbi Isaac Nissenbaum in the Warsaw Ghetto in the 1940s, is *Kiddush Ha-Hayim*, 'the sanctification of life', that is, one could and should defend one's soul against those who want to extinguish it—by taking one's life away from the oppressor. In that sense, *Kiddush Ha-Hayim* is *defiant suicide* rather than *despairing suicide*.

The Roman Jewish historian, Flavius Josephus, was the first to describe what has come to be called 'the Masada complex' (Josephus 1984 edn). Atop Herod's rocky citadel adjacent to the Dead Sea in Israel, the Jewish Zealots held out against the Roman army, but by 73 CE, it was clear they couldn't sustain the siege. Rather than submit to slavery or possible 'de-Judaising', 960 men, women and children took their lives. Regardless of the controversy about this 'complex'—that it is memorialised and celebrated as resistance by many and condemned as a form of cowardice by others—it is a tale of terrible choices and of a political and wilful act of response, of defiance in the face of the unthinkable, namely, the surrendering of their Jewishness.

Whether German Jews in the 1930s consciously thought about Masada is not known. But what is plain from the definitive analysis of historian Konrad Kwiet is that German Jewish suicide rates increased markedly in the Nazi era. There were two explanations of the escalation: first, suicide by those who had converted to Christianity, even as far back as two generations, when confronted by Nazi definitions of 'Jew' as anyone having at least one Jewish parent or one maternal or paternal grandparent. To be a devout Christian and a *Vaterland*-loving patriot and find oneself 'uncitizened' by the Nuremberg Laws of 1935, thus banished from public service of any kind, and then having to wear a yellow armband, was more than enough for some and they put an end to what they foresaw as an impossible life as a Jew under the Nazi regime. Then, there were those who, in a real sense, resisted the Nazis by taking their lives before the *Reich* took them. These Jews hoarded barbiturates over a longish period and, adjudging the time had come, found 'the ultimate refuge'. Remarkably, or perhaps not, wherever Nazis found Jews in a comatose or parlous state they saved them, in order to kill them in times and places of the Nazi choosing. Here, we see Lester's contention that victims seek freedom in death. It is also what the Hungarian-American psychiatrist Thomas Szasz called 'the fatal freedom' (Szasz 1998).

The Austrian essayist Jean Améry (1912–1978), who survived Auschwitz and Buchenwald, wrote agonising and acute analyses of the Holocaust, later a carefully considered book on suicide—and then ended his life. People, he contended, kill themselves out of a sense of dignity, preferring annihilation to the continuing existence lived in ignominy, or in desperate pain (physical or mental), or in utter helplessness (Améry 1999). Améry conceived of suicide not so much as an exit from life but as an entrance into another state, namely, death. [This was supported by the years of fieldwork among Australian Aboriginal societies when a number of Aboriginal parasuicides reported to Colin Tatz that they wanted to try it out 'up there' rather than remain in their present environs].

Foucault's concepts of biopower and biopolitic (Foucault 2003) and Barbagli's pairing are appropriate in the Australian Aboriginal context. The state exercises power over their body in a range of ways—from birth control practices, compulsory sterilisation, to vaccination regimens, to regulations protective of epidemics, prohibitions on circumcision, marriageable ages, multiple marriages, divorce, assisted dying and, as we have seen, suicide. The Nazi administration of life and, of course, death, was the ultimate example of total state control of the physical bodies in their domain.

7.4 Australia

The 2016 census enumerated the combined Aboriginal, Torres Strait Islander and South Sea Islander population as 649,200, or 2.8% of the (now 25 million) national population.[2] In northern Australia in the 1960s and 1970s, there was no record of any suicide in remote, rural or in urban communities—quite a contrast with suicide among Arctic Inuit and Indian peoples and New Zealand Māori.

'Ethnopsychiatry' was a research fad from 1960 to 1990, and several studies in the Northern Territory and Western Australia—by, among others, John Cawte (1968), Malcolm Kidson and Ivor Jones (1968), Ivor Jones (1973), P. W. Burvill (1975) and Harry Eastwell (1988)—found no 'mental health issues' and 'nothing alarming about Aboriginal suicide'. [Towards the end of the 1980s, Ernest Hunter began his pioneering work on Aboriginal history, health and suicide (Hunter 1988)]. Much of ethnopsychiatry in Australia was less about studying sorcery and native belief systems and much more about Western-perceived illness among the clans. This kind of ethnopsychiatry—always conducted on fleeting field visits, in [academic] English among solely dialect-speaking people (and sometimes by observing 'subjects' through binoculars at a distance)—was, for the most part, a dismal art, unproductive and without any portending quality. Nevertheless, we have to accept at face value the findings of these earlier researchers.

Our interest in suicide began in 1989–1990 when Colin Tatz explored the role of sport in deflecting Aboriginal juvenile delinquency (Tatz 1994). Conducted across 79 communities, this continent-wide fieldwork coincided with the appointment of a Royal Commission into Aboriginal Deaths in Custody, which established an investigation into 99 such deaths between 1980 and 1989 (RCIADC 1991). [There was a mistaken belief that most of these deaths were 'assisted' and highly suspicious—and

---

[2]New South Wales 216,176; Queensland 186,458; Western Australia 75,978; Northern Territory 58,248; Victoria 47,788; South Australia 34,184; Tasmania 23,572; Australian Capital Territory 6,508.

very few were. Noteworthy is that half of the custody deaths were of men who were of the 'stolen generations', that is, children forcibly removed from their natural parents.] He heard several stories of young deaths and young attempts, seemingly more common outside of custody than inside. So it proved to be.

Apart from a literal handful of cases, there was *no record* of Aboriginal suicides before 1960 (McIlvanie 1982), and suicide had no place in any Aboriginal belief systems, languages and material culture. Nor did Aboriginal suicide appear in prison, police or hospital records, in the files of children's institutions, in anthropologists' writings or notes, or in any missionary or governmental documents. Yet in the past 50–58 years their rates of suicide have soared to among the highest in the world, especially in the younger age groups—not just 15 to 24 but in the 10- to 14-year-old cohort. Lamentably, eight-year-olds are trying it, 'playing hangsies' as it is described in the Kimberley region of Western Australia. Even allowing for David Lester's comment (in the chapter headnote above) about American Indian [or Aboriginal] youth being inured to death at an early age, how does an eight year old, deemed in law not to have the capacity even to form *any* intent, then determine, understand, and act out self-cessation? Survivor children have articulated that they knew what death was. Such official statistics as we have told us that while the national suicide rate is now 12.6 per 100,000 of the population, for Aborigines and Torres Strait Islanders it is at the 24 per 100,000 level. In three states, the rate is closer to 30. For the years 1996 to 1998, rates of 40 were found in specific rural New South Wales Aboriginal communities (Tatz 2005: 59–69). In 2014, the Kimberley rate was 74. (The rural rate is higher than the urban figure.)

Aboriginal Suicide is Different: A Portrait of Life and Self-Destruction was first published in 2001 (Tatz 2001, 2005). Reactions varied: most were surprised or astonished, but one or two critics demanded to know how and in what ways Aboriginal suicide was, or could even remotely be considered 'different'. Academic psychologist Joseph Reser saw the 'differentness' as 'ostensible', 'rhetorical', with dangerous consequences for professional practice (Reser 2004). Wedded as they are to the axiom that an inexorable factor in suicide is previous suicide in families, Reser and others insisted that there simply had to be a history of Aboriginal suicide even in the absence of historical evidence. Psychiatry professor Robert Goldney chided Colin Tatz's failure to look at mental disorders in the suicides of two indigenous Taiwanese groups and in Han Chinese from the mainland (Goldney 2002).

In subsequent writings, and after research visits to New Zealand and Nunavut in Canada, the 'different' or varied quality was made clearer: one sharp look at the social, political and historic contexts revealed the divide. While suicide is suicide, the origins, social factors and the legacies of history make for a very different kind of analysis, the kind most health professionals are not exposed to. (In Chap. 12, we deal with the extent to which health professions are or aren't educated about suicide, let alone suicide as a social phenomenon.)

Aborigines trail a history like no other segment of the population, here or abroad. They experienced a genocidal era of episodic physical killings from 1804 to 1928, with some 150 massacre sites documented to date (Reynolds and Ryan 2017). Some 20,000 to 30,000 people were killed, by intent, in sporadic but systemic acts of 'dispersal' or 'dispersal of kangaroos' (as the official euphemism phrased it). To prevent the killings, federal and state governments (between 1897 and 1912) introduced policies of protection–segregation in the form of incarceration on isolated reservations. Between 1897 and the mid-1970s, governments sequestered between 70,000 and 90,000 people by erecting legal and geographic fences to preclude predators who sought to take the women and children and to sell them opium.

A reign of forcible child removal began in the late 1830s in colonial Victoria and lasted until the mid-1980s, with possibly 35,000 children affected. The aim was to eliminate Aboriginality by biological and social assimilation, by 'breeding out the colour', and by child re-acculturation, 'to erase them from the landscape' to the point, said officialdom, that no one would know that Aboriginal people ever existed (Haebich 2005: 267–289; Tatz 2011: 17–18). Throughout these phases, Aborigines had no civil or civic rights as generally understood: they were officially declared wards of the state, with government officials and Christian missionaries their legal guardians, irrespective of their age or ability to manage their own affairs (Tatz 2017; see McCorquodale 1987 for the details of statutory provisions controlling Aboriginal lives.)

Harsh as it was in terms of human rights and fundamental freedoms, the institutional era did maintain ordered communities. There were containable levels of physical violence, usually traditional methods of conflict resolution. But with the opening up of these near-prison-like regimes in the mid-1970s, disorder set in, with increasing deaths from non-natural causes. Officially called 'accidents and poisonings', this statistical category has, alarmingly, included high numbers and rates of homicide and suicide. [We accept Emanuel Marx's dictum that homicide is the flipside of suicide (Marx 1976)].

In the name of protection, nomadic hunter-gatherers had become sedentary, stationary, segregated as welfare recipients, pauperised in all walks of life. (There appears to be a link between suicide and abject poverty in several contexts.) The well-intentioned but draconian settlement and mission practices attempted to 'civilise' and Christianise them, to imbue them with notions of property, property ownership, aspiration, self-management. And then, suddenly, in the early 1970s, these governing authorities moved out and effectively abandoned them under the policy slogans of 'self-determination', then 'self-management' and then 'autonomy'.

The assaults on traditional culture thus occurred twice in less than 60 years. When the controlling authorities walked away, there was loss of both the traditional *and* the imposed structure, resulting in the trauma that Durkheim would call 'anomie'.

Johann Hari has written eloquently about 'lost connections' as the way to understand mental illness (Hari 2018) . The Aboriginal loss of connections has been calamitous, leading to many manifestations, including violence: loss of land, of life, of kin, children, language, traditional culture and ritual (often forbidden by statute), of freedom of movement, of a hunter-gathering lifestyle. They have experienced forcible relocation, loss of choice of living space. As recently as 2007, the conservative federal government introduced an 'intervention', ostensibly to quarantine Aborigines from excessive alcohol, drugs, sexual predators, and trespass from those deemed undesirable. This was essentially a reprise of the policies implemented in colonial Queensland in 1897: the strictest possible segregation and isolation but, in this instance, not to protect Aborigines from outside predators but from themselves. In sum, in the period of 230 years since White settlement in 1788, there have been massive impacts on Aboriginal lives: dispossession of land, massacres, isolation, strict segregation, forcible child removals, forced assimilation, fragmentation, denial of civic and civil rights, 'interventions' and, in more recent times, prison incarceration rates that are grossly excessive by any standards. Such are the contexts of 'difference'. [Public policies of equality, closing-the-gap and 'levelling the playing fields' don't like or appreciate these huge differences that need to be highlighted and accommodated: they get in the way of universality and expediency, two qualities precious to bureaucracies.]

Both Louis Wekstein's *Handbook of Suicidology* (1979) and Barbagli's book provide us with broad but definable genres and categories of suicide. Both acknowledge something society wants to avoid, namely, the very idea of *rational suicide*. There is no denying or relativising the reality that a percentage of the young who are bipolar, schizophrenic or experience severe mental disorders do commit suicide, but we are emphasising that the majority of suicides we have studied did not have such professionally diagnosed and confirmed mental illness. Nor do coronial files and witness depositions reveal presentations of that kind. A fair percentage of the remote population doesn't have regular, or even infrequent, contact with the professionals who can diagnose mental illness. As mentioned above, between 1960 and 1990 the major psychiatric studies found no evidence of *any* mental illnesses among Aborigines. Persons may have been unhappy, sad, grief-stricken, but they were neither clinically depressed nor unduly inclined to violence, to self or to others. An inability to cope with neo-liberal expectations and aspirations in modern society is not an illness as such. Often in rational ways—at least according to many interviews of the parasuicides, those who attempted suicide—they were not merely seeking an exit from life but, seemingly, an entrance to another state, a 'place' where life may possibly be better than the lives they have here, namely, death. Just as rationally, there are the many who reject our society and tell us so, more often than not by confrontational methods of death, like hanging in public places. In their own way, such public actions are political statements (Hunter 1988). Hanging (technically, asphyxiating) is hugely more prevalent than gun use, imbibing poison, jumping, train-surfing, drowning, self-immolating or climbing onto electricity power lines.

Two contextual factors loom large in the Aboriginal experience: their very short lives, forever confronted by young deaths and the legacies of a recent past and a never-certain present. A number of social indicators illustrate the gap between contemporary Aboriginal and non-Aboriginal life. One is life expectancy. Aboriginal males can expect to live to 67, some 11.5 years less than non-Aboriginal males. A recent book on Aboriginal sports achievers (Colin Tatz and Paul Tatz 2018) has an entry on the Rovers Football Club from Ceduna in South Australia, winners of a premiership in 1958. Of the eighteen young men in that Australian Rules football team,[3] only one lived to the age of 50. The Rovers team is a truer indicator of Aboriginal life (and death) than the numerical portrait provided by the Australian Bureau of Statistics.

During decades of fieldwork it was obvious enough that in most communities, there is at least one death, natural or unnatural, one funeral, one wake, every week. Children are inured to death at a very early age. Grief suffuses communities and the notion of grief counselling seems alien to all concerned. Horwitz and Wakefield (2007) lamented the 'loss of sadness' and the way psychiatry has turned sadness into a mental disorder. There is no shortage of sadness in Aboriginal life. Sadness is not clinical depression, and sadness is reason enough to end the body that is suffused by it.

An anecdote illustrates the point. In a remote western New South Wales town, Colin Tatz was asked to meet four young Aboriginal men who had attempted suicide and were heavily dosed with Prozac (the antidepressant). They took him to the cemetery, where they pointed to the grave of a 16-year-old once-promising footballer who had knocked down an old lady while trying to steal her purse and thought, wrongly, that he had killed her—whereupon he took a skipping rope from his gym bag and hanged himself in the public park. The four had bought a 24-can carton of beer: as they each drank a can, so they poured a matching one into the grave for Peter. Why are you doing that? 'We want to join him' was the unanimous and unambiguous reply. [In this story, we have a mix of loss, sadness, trauma, alcohol and antidepressants: yet we feel that loss and reconnecting were at the heart of their behaviour.]

The legacies of genocide on victim communities have barely been studied. We are beginning to comprehend the impacts on Armenian, Jewish, Bosnian and Rwandan communities. But what isn't recognised, or sufficiently recognised, is the impact beyond the second and third generations. Genocidal memory always lingers. It is osmosed down through to the descendants; it hovers in the background and often permeates and suffuses the foreground. It surrounds and invades life and is to be found in songs, stories, legends, attitudes to food, in art, language, idiom. And while youth may not know the details, they feel and embrace the emotions. One only has to ask an eight-year-old Armenian child, anywhere, what makes them Armenian and different, and they will refer to their genocide. There is, indeed, an ineluctable phenomenon that David Lester called tribal memory, an *understanding* memory rather than an *explanatory* memory.

---

[3] Australian football (sometimes called Australian Rules football, or Aussie Rules or plain 'footy'), is played over four quarters on an oval-shaped field, with eighteen players on each side. The ball is kicked or handled, forwards or backwards, and the object is to kick the ball through centre (or inner) goalposts for six points, and through adjoining side posts for one point. Non-fans have called it 'aerial ping-pong'.

Aborigines are among the world's best oral historians. In the space of some 180 years, six generations, they have endured genocidal massacres, culturally destructive incarceration on reserves, wholesale child removals and physical relocations, and then, in the name of autonomy with the arrival of Gough Whitlam's Labor Party government in 1972, the sudden removal of all infrastructure. However authoritarian, it left an ill-prepared mass to fend for themselves in isolation. Then came the Aboriginal 'intervention' by conservative Prime Minister John Howard of a decade ago and the re-infantilising of whole populations in the name of saving them from themselves. In short, five (rather than just two) dramatic onslaughts on a people in a very short historical time frame. Aboriginal suicide, unknown before 1960, irrupted savagely after that date, the dates that coincided roughly with so-called equal rights, civil rights and Aboriginal autonomy. Few ethnic communities have a history such as theirs and few remember their history the way they do.

Among the many flaws in the *DSM* dictionary of disorders, the disregard of grief is one of the most grievous. Grief, or bereavement, is normal, not a medical condition, or a condition that can be limited to a 'value' of two weeks or two months. Grief is not a fortnight's worth of tears, or a year-long sackcloth-and-ashes regimen found in some religions. Grief as in a formal funeral and an alcohol-fuelled wake may be the norm in Western Anglo societies but in many cultures mourning rituals are intrinsic to being (and dying). Much has been written about traditional Aboriginal mourning ceremonies and their significance. The present-day absence of those rites, and their lack of substitution, is a key factor in long-term grief, unresolved and unrequited grief. The grief of the Aboriginal quartet discussed above was manifesting a full two years after the footballer's suicide. What is unhelpful in all of these Aboriginal contexts is the particularly strident Australian penchant for an often inappropriate mantra—'move on'.

In the Aboriginal case—as with other ethnic minority victims—there is collective grief, a tone and tension that is diffused across a community. It isn't particularly difficult to comprehend what the German sociologist Ferdinand Tönnies termed *gemeinschaft*, commonly a tight-knit community of people with like tastes, values, attitudes and beliefs. Western society, urban society, with its more insular, privacy-seeking nuclear family structure, tends in such situations to grieve alone, or in tighter circles.

We have before us a remarkable catalogue of collective grief in a 1997 document, *Bringing Them Home* (HREOC 1997). After nearly two decades of Aboriginal agitation for an inquiry into the 'stolen generations' of Aboriginal children, a federal Labor Party government instituted an inquiry into 'the separation' of Aboriginal and Torres Strait Islander children from their families. The word 'separation' in the Commission's terms of reference was meant to infer that removal was temporary and a re-uniting was always in mind. It never was. The whole purport of the child removal policy was that 'transfer' would be permanent. The Inquiry heard 523 witness testimonies and came to the conclusion that genocide was, indeed, committed by the act of forcible transfer of children from one group to another group (as defined in Article II(e) of the UN Genocide Convention).

The essential themes of *Bringing Them Home* were grief and loss. The testimonies of the 'stolen' were, of course, gut-wrenching—endless tales of coercion, undue cruelty, physical and mental trauma while incarcerated in 'assimilation homes', constant sexual and physical abuse, humiliation, denigration, dehumanisation, often leading to attempts at harm to self.

Two short testimonies here illustrate the experiences. Rosalie Fraser (Tatz 2017: 118):

> The date was 13 March 1961, the place was Beverley in Western Australia. On that day my brother and sister, Terry aged eight, Stuart aged six, Karen aged four-and-a-half, Beverley aged eight months, and myself, were all made Wards of the State through action taken by the Child Welfare Department of Western Australia. The boy and girls were sent to separate institutions and Rosalie was later 'collected' by her foster mother, Mrs Kelly. When we first went to the Kellys, we had no idea where our parents were, we never saw or heard from them and we were unaware of what efforts they might be making to get us back. The Welfare communicated not with us but with the Kellys. The separation was total; our new life was the only one we knew.

Marjorie Woodrow was born in a small New South Wales country town. 'It was alleged that she had stole a pair of stockings'. Told that her mother was dead, she was sent to Cootamundra Girls' Training Home, one of the more notorious of many such institutions (Tatz 2017: 121):

> We were all Aboriginal, we were never called by our names. It was always 'number 108, step forward!' We had numbers sewn on our uniforms. Everyone could see that we were from the Girls' Home. We were branded just like cattle.

There is a thread that runs through child removal practices: grandmothers, daughters and daughters' daughters endured such institutional lives. We know several generations of women who have had that experience. It is not often that an Aboriginal youth experiences a one-off incarceration: the norm was and still is systematic and systemic.

In the aftermath of the Holocaust, the eminent neurologist and psychiatrist Viktor Frankl published *Man's Search for Meaning* (first published 1946). He wrote about those who survived [Nazi selections for death] but who nevertheless were beaten, starved, tortured. Survivors, he wrote, had a purpose in life. Another camp survivor, the Italian chemist Primo Levi, wrote much the same thing in his *The Drowned and the Saved* [*i sommersi e i salvati*] (Levi 1986). Reading Aboriginal testimonies, one can see, not always clearly but clearly enough, who were *salvati*, people determined to 'outlive' those who incarcerated and mistreated them, and those who drowned—by alcohol, drugs, violence to others or to selves.

7.5   Canada and the USA

The research literature on North American native peoples has grown remarkably in the past three decades. Andrew Woolford and Anthony Hall are leading the research into the genocidal aspects of Indian communities in North America, especially their impact on children who experienced the compulsory residential boarding schools (Woolford 2015; Hall 2018). The multidisciplinary scholar Michael Kral has been in the forefront of research into community participation in suicide prevention programmes in the Arctic (Kral 2019). Most scholars today have had the benefit of major investigations in Canada: the Royal Commission on Aboriginal People (1991–1996) and the Truth and Reconciliation of Canada Report of 2015 (Honouring the Truth 2015.) The latter gave voice to what had happened:

> Physical genocide is the mass killing of the members of a targeted group, and biological genocide is the destruction of the group's reproductive capacity. Cultural genocide is the destruction of those structures and practices that allow the group to continue as a group. States that engage in cultural genocide set out to destroy the political and social institutions of the targeted group. Land is seized, and populations are forcibly transferred and their movement is restricted. Languages are banned. Spiritual leaders are persecuted, spiritual practices are forbidden, and objects of spiritual value are confiscated and destroyed. And, most significantly to the issue at hand, families are disrupted to prevent the transmission of cultural values and identity from one generation to the next. In its dealing with Aboriginal people, Canada did all these things.

In 1994, the American Indian and Alaska Mental Health Research Center published the proceedings of a major conference. *Calling from the Rim* may well be the most important and coherent account of youth suicide among indigenous peoples. Dozens of medical and psychiatric journal papers cited quite diverse rates of Indian suicide within tribal groups, while others pointed to sharp differences in prevalence between tribes. (Canada, as a whole, has an Indian suicide rate of 38.4 as opposed to the national rate of 14.1.).

As discriminating as these studies appear to be, there remains the problem of the all-embracing title of 'tribe'. *Custer Died for your Sins* by Vine Deloria Jr, a well-known Indian rights advocate and a former Executive Director of the National Congress of American Indians, remains the most searing, and unrebutted indictment of American Indian policy, and of White academic attitudes, especially those of anthropologists. He deplored the Little Big Horn and wigwam stereotyping of his people, and while he has not written specifically about suicide, his admonitions of anthropology would apply as strongly to suicidology. In essence, he condemned academe for creating 'unreal' Indians in their attempts to establish 'real' Indians. Relevant here is Deloria's reminder that when academics talk of the Chippewas or the Sioux, they appear not to recognise that 'there are 19 different Chippewa tribes, 15 Sioux tribes, four Potawatomi tribes' and so on in Canada.

Anthropology may well have committed many 'sins' against Indian peoples. But the anthropological approach at least attempted to get to know 'their' people and 'their' tribes. Other social science and medical disciplines have adopted a distant, statistical approach, even where there are attempts at differentiation between reservation and non-reservation residents, as in a Manitoba study. There is no detail of historical experience or of lifestyle difference, only difference in geographic domain. In short, there is no context—social, historical, political—provided in these studies, apart from stating the inevitably obvious that these communities are impoverished, with high rates of unemployment, etc.

Every suicide study reports increasing numbers of attempts by females, but makes an important point that clustering is more common among females and that more females succeed in their purpose when among the cluster. Without being explicit, there is a strong message that female youth-attempted suicide is in need of serious attention.

Lester provides the best statistical summary of youth suicide, albeit with data at least a decade old. Despite regional differences, there is a sameness about many of the figures and ostensible causes. The 'indigenous' rates are said to be not three times but at least *ten times higher* than the national rates. The attempted suicides are vastly more prevalent.

Lester admitted the unreliability of standard psychology tests when used with Indians. His checklist of the 'standard' underlying factors is similar to the one in common use in Australia and New Zealand: depression, hopelessness, immaturity, aggressiveness, a history of suicidal behaviour, psychiatric problems, substance abuse, parent and family conflict, lack of family support, physical and sexual abuse and recent stress. He listed the sociological factors as social disintegration, cultural conflict and family breakdown. However, he added, 'rarely is cultural conflict listed among the precipitating causes'. It is not clear whether he was being critical of that omission or whether he, himself, believed it not to be significant. Yet his references to genocide were but fleeting, as in the chapter headnote quotation.

David Bechtold (1988) is one of the few researchers who talked about 'culturally sensitive risk factors' for males aged 12-plus. He didn't quite broach the legacies of such factors as the compulsory residential school era. Rather, he discussed physical and intellectual developmental precocity (12–14); conceptual maturity regarding death; conceptual familiarity with suicide through family or peer group or media exposure; substance abuse, depression, antisocial behaviour; previous suicide gestures and attempts; cultural mismatch between the youth and the environment; suicidogenic messages from family, especially parents; family disruption and dysfunction; and availability of lethal means. Our perspective was that many of these ingredients could well stem from the genocidal events.

Genocide produces many aftershocks. Loss is one, grief another. A third is pain, even chronic pain. For those living in the domains of the perpetrators, they know that they dwell among those who believed their values and/or their lives were not worth living. That is their baseline: the dysfunction, hopelessness, helplessness, despair, drugs, alcohol—aggression comes later. At-risk factors are but the overt expressions and symptoms of a deeper layer of pain and ways of dealing with it—physical, biological and cultural genocide.

References

American and Alaskan Native Mental Health Research Center. (1994). *Calling from the Rim: Suicidal behavior among American Indian and Alaskan Native adoles*cents, monograph series, volume 4, Journal of the National Center, Niwot, CO: University of Colorado Press.

Améry, J. (1999). *On suicide: A discourse on voluntary death.* Bloomington, IN: Indiana University Press.

Barbagli, M. (2015). *Farewell to the world: A history of suicide*, NJ: Wiley.

Burvill, P. W. (1975). Attempted suicide in the Perth statistical division 1971–1972. *Australian and New Zealand Journal of Psychiatry, 9*(4), 273–279.

Bechtold, D. (1988). Cluster suicide in American Indian adolescents. *American Indian and Alaska Native Mental Health Research, 1,* 26–35.

Cawte, J. et al. (1968). *Arafura, Aboriginal town: The medico-sociological expedition to Arnhem Land in 1968.* (unpublished typescript), restricted use, call number MS 483, AIATSIS, Canberra.

Dadrian, Vahakn. (1986). The role of Turkish physicians in the World War I genocide of Ottoman Armenians. *Holocaust and Genocide Studies Journal, 1*(2), 169–192.

Deloria, V.S. Jr. (1988). *Custer died for your Sins—An Indian Manifesto.* Norman, OK: University of Oklahoma Press.

Eastwell, H. (1988). The low risk of suicide among the *Yolngu* of the Northern Terrotory: The traditional Aboriginal pattern. *Medical Journal of Australia, 148*(7), 338–340.

Foucault, M. (2003). *Power: The essential Foucault: Selections from the essential works of Foucault, 1954–1984.* London: Penguin Books.

Frankl, V. (1984 ed.). *Man's search for meaning*, New York, NY: Washington Square Press.

Goldney, R. (2002). Is Aboriginal suicide different? A commentary on the work of Colin Tatz. *Psychiatry, Psychology and Law, 9*(2), 257–259.

Hall, A. (2018). A national or international crime? Canada's Indian residential schools and the Genocide convention. *Genocide Studies International, 20*(1).

Hari, J. (2018). *Lost connections: Uncovering the causes of depression—And unexpected solutions.* London: Bloomsbury Circus.

Hillman, J. (1997). *Suicide and the soul.* Woodcock, CN: Spring Publications.

Horwitz, A., & Wakefield, J. (2007). *The loss of sadness: How psychiatry transformed normal sorrow into depressive disorder.* New York: Oxford University Press.

HREOC [Human Rights and Equal Opportunity Commission]. (1997). *Bringing Them Home: Report of the national inquiry into the separation of Aboriginal and Torres Strait Islander children from their families.* Sydney: Human Rights and Equal Opportunity Commission.

Hunter, E. (1988). On Gordian knots and nooses: Aboriginal suicide in the Kimberly. *Australian and New Zealand Journal of Psychiatry, 22,* 264–271.

Hunter, E. (1989). Changing mortality patterns in the Kimberley region of Western Australia 1957–86: The impacts of deaths from external causes. *Aboriginal Health Information Bulletin II*, May.

Josephus (1984). *The Jewish War*, London: Penguin Books.

Kévorkian, R. (2011). *The Armenian genocide: A complete history.* London: I B Taurus.

Kidson, M., & Ivor, J. (1968). *Psychiatric disorder among Aborigines of the Austrlian Western Desert* (unpublished typescript), call number PMS 918, AIATSIS, Canberra.

Kral, M.J. (2019). *The return of the sun: Suicide and reclamation among Inuit of Arctic Canada.* Oxford University Press.

Kwiet, K. (1984). The ultimate refuge: Suicide in the Jewish community under the Nazis. In *Leo Baeck Institute Year Book XXIX,* London: Secker and Warberg.

Leenaars, A., Wenckstern, S., Dyck, R., Kral, M., & Bland, R. (1998). *Suicide in Canada.* Toronto: University of Toronto Press.

Lester, D. (1997). *Suicide in American Indians.* New York, NY: Nova Science Publishers.

Marx, E. (1976). *The social context of violent behaviour: A social study of an Israeli immigrant town,* London, Routledge: Kegan Paul.

McCorquodale, J. (1987). *Aborigines and the law: A digest.* Canberra: Aboriginal Studies Press.

McIlvanie, C. [Stafford] (1982). The responsibility of people. BA Honours dissertation, Politics Department, University of New England, Armidale, NSW.

Miller, D., & Touryan Miller, L. (1992). Women and children in the Armenian genocide. In Richard Hovanissian (Ed.), *The Armenian genocide: History, politics, ethics.* New York, NY: St Martin's Press.

Miller, D., & Touryan Miller, L. (1999). *Survivors: An oral history of the Armenian genocide.* Berkeley: University of California Press.

RCIADIC [*Royal Commission into Aboriginal Deaths in Custody*]. (1991). Commissioner Elliott Johnson QC, National Report 5 volumes, Canberra: Australian Government Publishing Service.

Reser, J. (2004). What does it mean to say that Aboriginal suicide is different? Differing cultures, accounts and idioms in the context of Indigenous youth suicide. *Australian Aboriginal Studies, 2,* 34–53.

Reynolds, H., & Ryan, L. (2017). Colonial Frontier Massacres in Australia, 1788–1930. https://c21ch.newcastle.edu.au/colonialmassacres.

Szasz, T. (1998). *Fatal Freedom: The ethics and politics of suicide.* Santa Barbara, CA: Praeger.

Tatz, C. (1994 April). *Aborigines: Sport, violence and survival,* CRC Project 18/1989, Canberra: Criminology Research Council.

Tatz, C. (2001, 2005). *Aboriginal suicide is different: A portrait of life and self-destruction.* Canberra: Aboriginal Studies Press.

Tatz, C. (2017). *Australia's unthinkable genocide.* Bloomington IN: Xlibris.

Chapter 8
The Preventionists

> ***Prevention****: the act of stopping something from happening or arising.*
>
> —Oxford English Dictionary

> *Suicide can be prevented, it just takes leadership and careful investment to make a meaningful change in this area.*
>
> —Mental Health Australia [https://mhaustralia.org/media-releases/australia-must-focus-preventing-suicide]

Abstract The origins of the prevention concept in the USA; a century of suicide prevention programmes; analyses of suicide statistics and the 'science' of prevention; identifying at-risk groups; differing approaches to prevention; unachievable targets for suicide reduction; examining prevention strategies in Eastern Europe, Japan and New Zealand.

Keywords Prevention · Statistics · World-wide comparisons

The concept of suicide prevention is more than a century old. This has been sufficient time in which to evaluate whether it is possible to stop people taking their own lives. Back in 1906, Harry Marsh Warren, an American Baptist minister, opened the first dedicated suicide prevention organisation, appropriately titled Save-A-Life League. Writing about Warren's mission, Miller et al. (2013) suggested Warren recognised early on the relationship between financial conditions and suicide, seeing self-death as an inability to cope with undesirable circumstances. A year later, General William Booth, the Methodist preacher who founded the Salvation Army, established the Anti-Suicide Bureau in Britain. It was described as 'giving sympathetic and sensible advice to desperate persons tempted to end their existence'.[1] Thereafter, suicide prevention agencies opened across Europe, with equally captivating names: the Advisory Centre

---

[1]Google. *The Bendigo Advertiser*, Monday January 7, 1907: 5.

© Springer Nature Switzerland AG 2019
C. Tatz and S. Tatz, *The Sealed Box of Suicide*,
https://doi.org/10.1007/978-3-030-28159-5_8

for the Weary of Life (Vienna), the Anti-Suicide League (Zurich) and the Suicides Aid Society (Berlin).

A century later, what began as quaintly named agencies providing advice and aiding those in dire straits has transformed into a network of government, private, and not-for-profit organisations across the world.[2] Working with great commitment, prevention agencies have had some success in saving lives. Surveying the worldwide picture over the last hundred plus years, we wonder whether their vision is misframed: suicide can never be *stopped* from happening. It can be prevented in particular circumstances, with some individuals 'saved', others alleviated by deferral or deflection, a matter we discuss in our final chapter.

8.1   Suicide Statistics

We need a picture of what prevention addresses, namely, the large annual global numbers of the deceased [see Appendix] and the unknown number—anything from nine to 25 times the fatal episodes—who don't complete their intention. Can the preventionists claim with any certainty that their specific actions saved the non-completers?

In management, there is a saying that what gets measured gets done. Measuring suicide rates, however imprecisely, at least establishes broad trends and provides insight into countries with high suicide rates. In Chap. 6, we asked whether prevention can ever be a catch-all strategy for the many suicide categories and whether the prevention blueprints are designed for specific genres and kinds of suicide (and specific means). World-wide, according to the World Health Organization, someone ends their life every 40 seconds. How many attempt suicide is much harder to estimate. For the 15–29-year cohort, suicide is the second leading cause of death globally (WHO 2014). It isn't possible to determine how many of these suicides are by persons labelled as 'at risk'.

The Organisation for Economic Co-operation and Development (OECD) explained that data comparability is affected by a number of reporting criteria, with caution needed in 'interpreting variations across countries'. Suicide data rates are age-standardised to the 2010 OECD population.[3] The OECD table for suicide rates showed seven of the top 10 nations as Eastern European: Lithuania, Slovenia, Russia, Latvia, Hungry, Estonia and Poland (almost level with the USA). Countries engaged in war, civil strife and/or with high murder rates—South Africa, Mexico, Colombia,

---

[2]In Australia in 2016–2017, suicide prevention-specific programmes expended $A49.2 million out of a total of $A3 billion spent by the federal government on mental health. States probably spent about the same amount, so prevention expenditure was some $A100 million out of $8.7 billion. We think this is a major slab of money; others in this field believe it is far too little.

[3]Sourced from https://data.oecd.org/healthstat/suicide-rates.htm.

Israel and Brazil—have low suicide rates. Countries with high murder rates don't even appear on the OECD table. South Africa's current murder rate is 34.27 per 100,000 of the population, the seventh leading country for homicides, yet its suicide rate is just 1.0. Brazil and Mexico have high murder rates, but sit in the bottom 10 OECD nations for suicide. The USA has the tenth highest suicide rate, but the homicide rate is one-third of its suicide rate. Lithuania and Latvia are low on the murder 'league table' for homicides, yet both are in the top five for suicide. Wealthy Western and Asian nations—Belgium, Finland, USA, Australia, New Zealand, Sweden, Germany, Denmark, South Korea and Japan—have higher suicide rates than poorer Costa Rica, Turkey, Greece and Chile.

The quality and utility of statistics vary and need caution, if not scepticism. But they should give prevention agencies a rough idea of how to align their programmes with official suicide rates—which could well be double or even triple the official homicide rate. [There are no agencies, not even police forces, dedicated to thwarting homicide.]

8.2 Prevention is not a Science

In health, *prevention* means intervening before adverse effects set in. Routine immunisation, screenings and scans are integral to preventive health. 'Intervention' is to intercede in, to modify, even avert, an outcome. Medical evaluations are used to determine outcome criteria, assessing the effectiveness and value of a treatment. As discussed earlier, suicide is locked into the biomedical environment, guarded and guided by the helping professions. Evaluating preventions and interventions (we use the term preventions from here on) should, at least in theory, use similar tools of measurement. But suicide isn't cancer showing on a scan; it isn't a blood disorder or a genetic abnormality amenable to examination or verification.

How will the medical world (rather than the realm of the psychology and social work preventionists) view current suicide prevention practices a century hence? Will 'preventionists' abjure the overuse of antidepressants, the reliance on helplines, websites, apps and Facebook sites, and the millions expended on awareness-raising campaigns? Will they wonder why we were using approaches first initiated in 1906? Two centuries after the Save-A-Life League opened its doors, will we still be ignoring the social contexts of diverse forms of self-destruction?

We see much of preventionism as a way of forestalling blame, avoiding 'failure' to stop an 'epidemic'. Rarely questioned is the very notion of whether suicide can be prevented: the premise is that it can be and therefore it must be. Like other aspects of medicine, degrees of faith are required. Medical science has limits; the public accept that we cannot explain why some treatments work and others don't, that some diseases are incurable. Modern anaesthesia dates from 1842, and yet we don't fully understand the mechanisms by which it works. Today, the medical profession is grappling with cannabis and whether there is sufficient 'evidence' as opposed to 'observation' to prove its efficacy as a front-line treatment for seizures, and the like. Scientific verification and evaluation create an accountability that we hope, or assume, accompany a product to the market place. There are, of course, infamous exceptions, as with Prozac, discussed earlier.

Suicide prevention strategies have limits. In the absence of scientific protocols and clinical trials evaluating outcome criteria, an element of belief underpins the process. If suicide is a disease or disorder, if indeed there is a definable 'suicide' gene, then the preventions adopted should be open to evaluation, a matter discussed in the next chapter. A disconnect exists in prevention: while mental health professionals see suicide within medical parameters, prevention analyses are shapeless and fuzzy. Many strategies are not evaluated and those that are rarely publish the results of a review. Their focus is on outputs, not outcomes; which is why measuring the extent and recognition of awareness-raising material, counting the 'hits' on websites and apps, and calls to hotlines, substitutes for evidence. In Australia, more rigorous evaluation (particularly with Aboriginal and Torres Strait Islander suicide projects) is occurring (Jorm et al. 2012; ATSI SP 2017). But in our experience, the Jorm et al. study is correct: there is an inequality between Aboriginal and non-Aboriginal mental health services. The former is given less support than large-scale 'awareness' campaigns such as R U OK?—a national suicide prevention initiative based on 'starting a conversation'.

This is an understandable reaction. When a family member or friend ends a life, a passion to prevent others going through the same trauma is natural. Suicides cripple the living. Bereavement, loss and unanswered questions drive families, governments and mental health agencies for answers, efforts that should not be dismissed. These efforts have value, and we are not suggesting they don't save some lives; but we don't know to what extent prevention programmes are working, why they work in some regions and not others, why suicide rates fluctuate so widely within countries and between neighbouring countries, and why, after decades of trying and billions of dollars spent, suicide rates globally have not been reduced in any meaningful way. We don't even know what types of suicides the preventionists are trying to prevent. The distressed White, urban-dwelling teenager who rings for help at midnight is one end of the spectrum. But what can anyone do about the lonely, isolated elderly man or woman, the pensioner who is no longer able or allowed to contribute, the financier who has lost it all, the young lass who thinks she is fat, the sheep farmer surrounded by his thirst-dead animals?

8.3 Suicide and 'At-risk' Groups

Suicide rarely bleeps a warning. Instead, we turn to 'at-risk' factors as a way of detecting potential actors. That is as 'scientific' as Alphonse Bertillon's nineteenth-century system of measuring humans to ascertain who was likely to be a criminal, or modern police relying on 'racial profiling' to detect illegal behaviour. It is fraught with generalisations and assumptions; it takes an amorphous cohort of individuals and assigns them characteristics suggesting suicidality.

Certain individuals *are* 'at risk': those who have attempted suicide or expressed suicidal tendencies, those in custody and in mental health psychiatric wards. Standard protocol tests for patients/inmates are not conclusive but can be indicative in some way. Suicide watch protocols are relevant to prevention. Looking at one Australian jurisdiction (NSW), the *Protocols* stress not only whether suicidal plans have been expressed, but 'other' personal risk factors including recent major life events especially involving loss or humiliation; and 'at-risk' mental states related to hopelessness, despair, agitation, anxiety, shame, guilt, anger and psychosis.[4] Protective factors designed to prevent suicide include: 'strong perceived social supports; family cohesion; peer group affiliation; good coping and problem-solving skills; positive values and beliefs; [and] ability to seek and access help'. These 'protective factors' read more like a checklist for good mental health and resilience.

To prevent suicides, psychiatric units, prisons and custodial facilities routinely remove inmates/patients clothing and possessions, dress them in tear-proof or paper clothing and leave them in a locked 'suicide-proof' prison cell. Professor Christine Tartaro, an expert on suicide in correctional facilities, told CNN: 'Suicide watch has wound up being an incredibly bleak environment. There's not going to be a thing in there to help you take your mind off of that. It doesn't bode well for you being able to get better' (Tartaro 2017). CNN reported that suicides accounted for 7% of deaths in American state prisons (in 2014), while suicide rates in local county jails are 'more than twice that'.

Once the suicide is deemed 'prevented', psychiatric hospital patients are routinely released without post-discharge supports, housing or income. The high rates of suicide post-discharge may be a consequence of this, together with antiquated and inhumane incarceration and sedation. Writing in *JAMA Psychiatry*, Chung et al. (2017) confirmed high rates of suicide following discharge from 'psychiatric hospitalisation'. The post-discharge suicide rate for people admitted to psychiatric facilities was 'approximately 100 times the global rate during the first 3 months after discharge and patients admitted with suicidal thoughts or behaviours had rates near 200 times the global rate'. In the past 50 years, the rate of suicide for patients discharged from clinical institutions designed to prevent suicide through advanced psychiatric and

---

[4]Suicide Risk Assessment and Management Protocols: Mental Health In-Patient Unit NSW Health. See: www.health.nsw.gov.au/mentalhealth/programs/mh/Publications/mental-health-in-patient-unit.pdf.

medical care has not decreased. The authors fittingly commented: 'This is a disturbing finding considering the increase in community psychiatry and the availability of a range of new treatments during this period'. Psychiatrists treating patients admitted into clinical and acute hospital facilities cannot prevent suicide. It makes us question whether psychiatric units and hospitalisation are even the most appropriate place to 'secure' those exhibiting suicidal behaviour.

8.4   Problems with 'At-risk' Groups

Within the confines of prisons and secured hospital psychiatric units, suicides among those identified 'at risk' cannot be prevented. Within the general population, the U.S. Department of Health and Human Services has identified ten groups that 'have demonstrated a higher risk for suicide or suicide attempts'[5]:

- Lesbian, gay, bisexual or transgender persons (LGBT);

- military and veterans;

- those with mental disorders or substance-use disorders;

- American Indians and Alaska Natives;

- persons bereaved by suicide;

- those in justice and child welfare settings;

- persons who intentionally hurt themselves (non-suicidal self-injury);

- those who have previously attempted suicide;

- the medically ill; and

- men in midlife and older men.

Over 10 million Americans (4.1%) identify as LGBT. An estimated 20 million are military veterans.[6] Over 18% of adults or more than 43 million people struggle with mental health every year. Americans reporting a drug or alcohol problem account for 8.4% of the population, while 3.94% (9.4 million) individuals have suicidal thoughts.[7] American Indians and Native Alaskans number 6.7 million. When President Donald Trump wound back what was known as 'Obama Care' (*Afford-*

---

[5]The Substance Abuse and Mental Health Services Administration (SAMHSA) https://www.samhsa.gov/suicide-prevention/at-risk-populations.

[6]http://www.pewresearch.org/fact-tank/2017/11/10/the-changing-face-of-americas-veteran-population/.

[7]See: http://www.mentalhealthamerica.net/issues/2017-state-mental-health-america-prevalence-data.

able Care Act), an estimated 130 million non-elderly Americans had a pre-existing medical condition. Only halfway through the 'at-risk' groups the authors calculate 200 million 'at-risk' Americans in need of suicide prevention. Labelling of this kind is not helpful. A paradox emerges: mental health experts warn about the problems of stigma associated with suicide and help-seeking, yet they literally lump every homosexual, soldier, drug user, chronically ill or First Nations persons as a suicide risk.

In Australia, the government-initiated Mindframe has a similar list. A back of the envelope calculation highlights the problem with the Mindframe cohort: about 5 million in a population of 25 million are a suicide risk. In Australia, mere 'Aboriginality' is listed as a risk. The British Office for National Statistics (ONS) takes a much more reasoned approach. Divorce and socio-economics are risk factors, stressing these factors as only part of the reasoning.[8] What the ONS does well is provide explanations as to why men are mostly a suicide risk. They refer to research deciphering how men experience (and handle) different complexities, including family and relationship breakdowns and changing expectations about masculinity; for example, divorced men are almost three times more likely to exit than men who are married or in a relationship.[9] Identifying particular circumstances and life situations seems an eminently more logical and reasoned prevention approach. 'Situational suicide' best described circumstances accounting for male suicide (Ashfield et al. 2017). The situational approach posited suicide with a wider range of non-medical distressing factors, for example men in their 30s and 40s suddenly adrift from their partner (and children), socially isolated and either in poorly paid jobs or with skills no longer in demand or valued, end their lives not necessarily because of any treatable clinical mental health problems—they exit because they see no future and no value in their lives.

Innovative research by Ashfield et al. (2017) also perceived the suicide prevention focus on mental illness and disorder as 'problematical'. After listing a spectrum of situational distress factors (sickness, unemployment, financial difficulties, relationship breakdowns, bereavement, drug and alcohol issues, conflict, and trauma), they proposed that 'limiting prevention strategies to those built upon the unfounded presumption of mental illness or disorder will simply not help many, perhaps the majority, of those at risk of suicide' (Ashfield et al. 2017).

Labelling people is fraught with complications and may even contribute to suicidal tendencies. Does it follow that if you're told often enough that you are a suicide risk then perhaps one day that may be acted out?

---

[8]https://visual.ons.gov.uk/who-is-most-at-risk-of-suicide/.

[9]https://visual.ons.gov.uk/who-is-most-at-risk-of-suicide/.

8.5 Different Approaches to Prevention

We cannot evaluate every global suicide prevention programme. Certainly, some preventions achieve reductions in rates of suicide, others fluctuate in outcomes. As year in and year out figures shift without any evident longer-term trends, we've chosen examples from selected countries to highlight how factors other than mental illness contribute to suicide, and how these same factors (economics, stability, employment, agency and hope) can reduce suicide.

8.5.1 Suicide in Eastern Europe

Between 1990 and 2017 Lithuania, Latvia and Estonia—former states of the USSR— recorded the highest rates in the world. OECD statistics showed the Lithuanian rate had fluctuated from 28.6 per 100,000 in 1990 to 50.00 just five years later. Lithuania, a predominantly Catholic country (77% adherence), had seen suicide rates rise and fall dramatically. Professor Danute Gailiene from Vilnius University explained why: 'Suicide did not exist during the Soviet time because it did not fit the idea of a nation living happily under socialism … The word 'suicide' did not even appear in Soviet encyclopedias' (Sander 2015). Health researcher Antanas Grizas (Sander 2015) supported the view that Lithuania's high rates could be attributed to the Soviet-era medical approach. For Grizas, 'the biomedical approach to mental health problems still dominates' and little has changed since the Soviet era: 'We lack community-based approaches, social integration, as well as accessibility to psychological treatment'.

Suicide in former republics of the Soviet Union is a consequence of the massive upheavals that occurred pre- and post-World War II. An informative article with the rather odd title, 'Stalin, rock music and bad weather: story behind suicides in Lithuania' (Barro 2010), offered other reasons why this nation had so many suicides. Lithuania suffered badly during and after World War II. The Germans killed 90% of the Jewish population and then in 1944, the Soviets captured the country, a fate that befell other European nations. The population was traumatised and transformed. The massive increase in suicide wasn't the result of an epidemic of mental illness, but a consequence of social determinants of health—housing, poverty, substance abuse and massive political turmoil.

Alvydas Navickas, president of the Lithuanian Association of Suicidology and deputy head of psychiatry at the University of Vilnius, said the impact of World War II and Stalinism created a perfect storm for suicide. Lithuania was transformed from a mostly rural, religious society, with a strong sense of community and stable customs. When the Soviet Union seized control, they deported the wealthiest farmers to Siberia; those left behind were forced into *kolkhozes* (collective farms). 'Vodka and home-brewed alcohol began to flow like a daily anaesthetic' (Barro 2010). Before the

War, eight in 100,000 Lithuanians committed suicide each year; by the mid-1990s the rate was 46. Lithuanians taking their own lives were predominantly rural. As Navickas made clear, 'The only new thing independence brought to rural Lithuania was unemployment. Everything else is the same: poor infrastructure, a lack of social services, alcoholism…' The statistics are stark: about 30% of Lithuanians live in rural communities with poverty levels three times higher than in cities. Only half the population has showers (only 25% have running water) or indoor toilets. A European Commission study (2008) found high rates of poverty and a mass exodus from rural to urban centres. The upheavals in Lithuania left hundreds of thousands abandoned. As one young Lithuanian put it, 'We have nothing, there's no point working the land. People are killing themselves' (Barro 2010). This is situational suicide.

Lithuania only recently introduced suicide prevention strategies. At the time of writing, indications suggest the rate is declining, although it is not clear whether this is a consequence of these strategies or as a result of improved economic circumstances and employment opportunities or increased access to mental health services. Plain enough is that upheavals in Eastern Europe—along with transformations in their societal structures, governance, employment and social determinants—are a significant factor in their high rates of suicide.

An informative analysis by Pray et al. (2013) examined the variations in suicide in Eastern European nations, after a 2010 conference which discussed the evidence base for social and public health determinants of suicide. Their hypothesis was that the 'changes to societal transformations associated with the breakdown of the Eastern Bloc' accounted for why this region had the highest rates of suicide globally. Unlike most other conferences on suicide, mental illness was not the focus or even a major consideration. The themes explored showed a refreshing approach to suicide through the examination of culture, beliefs, religion, rural–urban divides, alcohol, financial and socio-economic standing, and the transformations of civil society. 'Depression' was listed as the very last topic discussed, and fittingly only accounted for 115 words with a brief, almost passing reference that depression can be the result of other underlying social determinants such as unemployment (Pray et al. 2013). Of particular interest was the emphasis given to alcohol consumption, which was described as a substantial determinant of suicidal behaviour. Even when considering differences in methodology, geography and culture, they found firm evidence for suicide prevention strategies to be developed around alcohol control. About 70% of suicides in Lithuania were alcohol related.

While mainstream psychiatric treatments for depression did not reduce suicide measurably, it was pointed out that alcohol control strategies had been successful in reducing alcohol-related mortality.

Lithuania is not an isolated example. Suicide is the second leading external cause of death in Belarus, another former Soviet state. Again, we see wide variations in suicide rates align with the massive transformations, including the relatively liberal *perestroika* period, which led many to believe the Soviet Union was becoming a more open and hopeful society. When these hopes crumbled with the collapse of the USSR, suicide rates increased. The seismic jolt created by the break-up of the paternalistic Soviet system produced a psychosocial distress that 'was the main determinant of the general suicide mortality crisis that swept across the former Soviet republics in the 1990s' (Pray et al. 2013).

The dean of the School of Criminal Justice at the State University of New York at Albany, William Alex Pridemore, said the turbulent and violent history of the Soviet Union had contributed to suicide and 'a bleak outlook on the future'. Alcohol played a crucial role in Russia and other Slavic nations, said Pridemore, where men were prone to high rates of binge drinking, especially vodka. The effects of distilled spirits 'can make people more likely to act on suicidal thoughts as well as indirectly contribute to mental health issues associated with economic hardship, domestic violence and family breakdown' (Watkins 2017). Similarly, Ukraine experienced a massive increase in suicides following independence in 1991. Consistent with its neighbours, the rise in suicide mortality was attributed to a combination of dire economic conditions and a hasty deterioration in the quality of life. For Ukrainians, the impact was in their industrial heartland and high-density regions. Suicide was linked to economic fluctuations with decreases in suicide mortality attributed to rising standards of living (Watkins 2017).

The analysis of suicide preventions in Eastern Europe is scant. Only in recent times have suicide prevention programmes been funded and rolled out. How widespread these are is not evident; however, a few conclusions can be drawn. Trauma on a massive scale has left many people in despair and without control of their lives or futures. Alcohol abuse was rampant. As a result, suicides skyrocketed. Improving economic circumstances following the break-up of the Soviet Union has now decreased rates.

8.5.2 Suicide in Japan

Japan's history, societal structures, beliefs, religion and culture are in almost every respect the opposite of Eastern Europe. And yet Japan has one of the highest—and most consistent—suicide rates in the world. Between 1990 and 2013, Japan's rate was remarkably consistent, although there has been a decrease in recent years. In 2015, National Police Agency statistics showed that 24,025 people killed themselves. In 1998, the number of suicides was 32,863. The rate was not attributed to mental illness but 'a surge in suicides, mostly among middle-aged men, due to joblessness linked to the bankruptcies of corporate behemoths' (Osaki 2016). Again, this is 'situational suicide', the ending of one's life based on what appears to be hopelessness, financial distress and quite likely loneliness and/or social isolation.

Japan's unique, highly regulated and structured culture is more a determinant of suicide than an alternative theory—that Japan has higher rates of mental illness which accounts for its high rates of suicide. In January 2018, the *Japan Times*[10] reported that suicides fell for an eighth consecutive year in 2017, dropping 3.5% from the previous year to 21,140; although there was an increase in youth suicide. *Japan Times* referred to Japan's recently adopted suicide prevention plan that set a target of reducing the ratio from 18.5 (in 2015) to 13.00 (by 2025). The plan, said the *Times*, aimed to address 'excessive working hours [and] prejudice against sexual minorities' along with postpartum depression. Japan's high rate, especially among men, correlated with employment. Their suicide prevention programmes include counselling services in employment agencies, and assistance in finding accommodation. Adachi official Yuko Baba, chief of the Mental and Physical Health Promotion Section, acknowledged that '[I]n many cases, those who committed suicide are those who desperately wanted to live. They decided to kill themselves because they couldn't live the way they wanted to (Osaki 2016)'.

Suicide has traditionally been a taboo topic for the Japanese people. It was seldom part of the public discourse. This changed in the mid-2000s when the unmentionable was brought into the open as a social problem.[11] The language is significant—suicide was to be considered a social problem, not a mental illness. In 2006, members of Japan's House of Councillors produced the *Basic Act for Suicide Prevention* (it became law in June 2006), an act enshrining preventing suicide as 'an overarching government policy not limited to any single ministry'. Prevention was based on addressing financial stress, not mental disorders. Interestingly, in 2016 Japan's national suicide prevention project was transferred from the Cabinet Office to the Ministry of Health, Labor and Welfare: a ministry that encompasses employment, primary health care and welfare seems ideally suited to understanding the many factors in suicide. Significantly, Japan experienced an increase in suicide during the global financial crisis.

In 2013, Japan initiated the Council for Evaluation on Suicide Prevention Programmes to see if their strategy was working as intended. One evaluation noted the need for longer-term studies to determine the effectiveness of the Japanese approach. Nakanishi et al. (2015) studied the effectiveness of Japan's national suicide fund, established following the release of 'General Principles of Suicide Prevention Policy' in 2007. Not every Japanese prefecture adopted the same measures, and it appears standardised programmes and accompanying workforce availability made evaluation difficult, but what the authors concluded is similar to other suicide prevention evaluations:

> However, the sole implementation of 'public awareness campaigns' exhibited no significant differences in systems for suicide prevention compared with those that did not implement any suicide-prevention programmes. As expected by the Council for Evaluation on Suicide

---

[10] 'Suicides in Japan notched eight consecutive drops in 2017, preliminary data show', January 19, 2018. https://www.japantimes.co.jp/news/2018/01/19/national/suicides-japan-notched-eight-consecutive-drop-2017-preliminary-data-show/#.WnEzNqiWaUk.

[11] 'Japan turning the corner in suicide prevention' in http://www.who.int/mental_health/suicide-prevention/japan_story/en/

Prevention Programmes, there was no significant association between suicide rates during the 4-year period and the implementation of suicide-prevention programmes. One literature review suggested that short duration interventions may have limited effects on suicide rates.

8.5.3 New Zealand

Professor Sir Peter Gluckman, the chief science adviser in New Zealand's Office of the Prime Minister, in a paper on youth suicide, began by making the point that youth suicide in New Zealand is 'more than simply a mental health issue'. He focussed on primary prevention and early life, and described the context and pressures young New Zealanders face: changes to family structures and child-rearing customs, the ways technology and social media have transformed communications (and interpersonal relationships), the expectations and pressures placed on young people, and the decline in structured societal entities, such as religious organisations, sport and even youth activities. None of these characteristics are unique to New Zealand.

The data cited by Gluckman et al. showed that, in 2010, New Zealand's youth suicide mortality rate was 15.6 per 100,000 (adolescents aged 15 to 19 years), a figure the authors say is the highest in the OECD. For Māori youth, the suicide mortality rate (15 to 24 years) was 48.0 per 100,000 in 2012. And while youth suicide rates have declined for non-Māori, young Māori youth continue to have higher rates of suicide and self-harm. Youth suicide in New Zealand is attributed to a number of factors that align with general social determinants of health: poverty, inequality, high rates of substance abuse, interaction with the police and the criminal justice system, and social fragmentation. Gluckman added other factors that are germane to indigenous youth: 'living in environments where low self-esteem within the peer group is common [and] suicidal behaviour becoming a means of demonstrating worth to the peer group'. In a pattern we are seeing across much of the literature, the New Zealand analyses reveal the links between alcohol misuse/abuse and suicide, especially in men. On mental health and youth suicide, the paper described:

> the challenge of differentiating mental illness as a cause of suicide in young people from depression as an associated symptom of disorganised brain, biological, social and behavioural development. Although cognitive behavioural therapy (CBT) is effective in treating depression in adolescents, it does not reliably reduce the risk of suicidal attempts … In general, psychotherapy appears to be only marginally helpful in reducing suicide. The use of antidepressant pharmaceuticals appears to be no more effective than CBT in preventing suicide (Gluckman 2017:8).

Addressing New Zealand's approach to prevention, the authors stressed primary prevention, beginning at pre-pubescence, which develops resilience and improves educational and employment outcomes. Alcohol reduction is listed as a primary prevention. As for other suicide prevention approaches (in schools), 'it is less clear' whether these are effective 'except in reducing contagion. Indeed, some programmes may actually increase the risk of suicidality, hence the importance of oversight and formal evaluation of all such programmes'. Programmes that promote 'economic development in disadvantaged communities' and 'promoting community self-worth' are among the main social investments that act as suicide prevention. The conclusion was direct: 'A focus on adolescent mental health, although important, is not sufficient'.

New Zealand's suicide prevention strategies target both indigenous and non-indigenous people. It wasn't until the mid-2000s that the New Zealand government implemented a national suicide prevention strategy. From the look of it, their approach was to limit access to suicide 'hot spots' such as well-known bridges (Australia has a similar programme) and trying to decrease access to weapons.

Over 100 years ago, Harry Marsh Warren, 'a largely forgotten figure' (Miller et al. 2013), founded the first suicide prevention agency. In an era before antidepressants, DSMs and medical interventions, Warren offered more than sympathetic counselling for the suicidal; he provided free accommodation and legal services, material goods for the destitute, for he believed economic circumstances and value influenced suiciders; his volunteers supported families; he championed health care over prison for those he thought were mentally unwell.

We ask, how far has the preventionists approach advanced in the century since the Save-A-Life League began?

References

Ashfield, J., Macdonald, J., Francis, A., & Smith A. (2017). A *"situational approach" to mental health literacy in Australia*. May, University of Western Sydney paper.

ATSI SP. (2017). *Report of the Critical Response Pilot Project, Aboriginal and Torres Strait Islander Suicide Prevention Evaluation Project*, July.

Barro, A. (2010). Stalin, rock music and bad weather: story behind suicides in Lithuania. Café Babel, May 17, 2010. www.cafebabel.co.uk/culture/article/stalin-rock-music-and-bad-weather-story-behind-suicides-in-lithuania.html.

Chung, D. T., Ryan, C. J., Hadzi-Pavlovic, D., Singh, S., Stanton, C., & Large, M. (2017). Suicide rates after discharge from psychiatric facilities; a systematic review and meta-analysis. *JAMA Psychiatry, 74*(7), 694–702. https://doi.org/10.1001/jamapsychiatry.2017.1044.

European Commission. (2008). *Poverty and social exclusion in rural areas*, European Commission. Directorate-General for Employment, Social Affairs and Equal Opportunities.

Gluckman, S. P. (2017). *Youth Suicide in New Zealand: A Discussion Paper*. 26 July. Prepared by Sir Peter Gluckman in conjunction with the Departmental Science Advisors from the Ministries of Heath (Prof J. Potter), Education (Prof. S. McNaughton), Justice (Prof I. Lambie) and Social Development (Prof R Poulton).

Jorm, A., Bourchier, S. J., Cvetkovski S., & Stewart G. (2012). Mental health of indigenous Australians: A review of findings from community surveys. *Medical Journal of Australia, 196*(2), 118–121. https://doi.org/10.5694/mja11.10041. Published online: February 6, 2012.

Miller, D. N. & Gould K. (2013). *Forgotten founder: Harry Marsh Warren and the history and legacy of the Save-A-Life League*. University at Albany, State University of New York, USA. Suicidology Online 2013; 4:12–15. http://www.suicidology-online.com/pdf/SOL-2013-4-12-15.pdf.

Nakanishi, M., Yamauchi, T., & Takeshima, T. (2015). National strategy for suicide prevention in Japan: Impact of a national fund on progress of developing systems for suicide prevention and implementing initiatives among local authorities (2014, August) in *Psychiatric and Clinical Neurosciences, 69*(1), 5–64. January 2015.

Osaki, T. (2016). Landmark new laws put suicide prevention front and center. *Japan Times*, March 30, 2016. https://www.japantimes.co.jp/news/2016/03/30/national/social-issues/landmark-new-laws-put-suicide-prevention-front-center/#.WnFRvaiWaUk.

Pray, L., Cohen, C., Mäkinen, I. H., Värnik A., & MacKellar L. (Eds.). (2013). Suicide in Eastern Europe, the CIS, and the Baltic Countries: Social and Public Health Determinants. A Foundation for Designing Interventions Summary of a Conference. International Institute for Applied Systems Analysis ZVR-Nr: 524808900. RR-13-001. February 2013. http://suicidology.ee/wp-content/uploads/2016/10/Suicides-in-Eastern-Europe-RR-13-001-web.pdf.

Sander, G. (2015). Lithuania looks to shed unwelcome distinction: suicide capital of Europe. *Christian Science* Monitor. 19 November www.csmonitor.com/World/Europe/2015/1119/Lithuania-looks-to-shed-unwelcome-distinction-suicide-capital-of-Europe.

Tartaro, C. (2017). CNN interview. https://edition.cnn.com/2017/04/19/health/suicide-watch-prevention/index.html.

Watkins, J. (2017). Story behind Russia's male suicide problem. *The Daily Dose*. www.ozy.com/acumen/the-story-behind-russias-male-suicide-problem/76845.

WHO. (2014). *Preventing suicide: A global imperative*. World Health Organisation. ISBN 978 92 4 156477 9 (NLM classification: HV 6545). Library Cataloguing-in-Publication Data.

Chapter 9
The Evaluators

To evaluate: to ascertain the value of, to appraise carefully.

To review: a looking over or an examination with a view to amendment or improvement.

—Webster's New International Dictionary

There is no single suicide prevention program that appears to be effective in reducing suicide rates.

—Prevention Strategies: Evidence from Systematic Reviews (Guo et al. 2003)

Abstract Questioning the criteria by which suicide prevention strategies are assessed for their quality and their achievements; how to evaluate suicide prevention strategies and policies; observational outputs versus evidence-based outcomes; paucity of review of suicide prevention in Australia; what is achieved by awareness-raising and anti-stigma campaigns?

Keywords Appraisals · Feedback · Lessons learned

Good Samaritan laws (and agencies) offer assistance to those in peril, dire need or who are suffering serious injury. Soup-kitchens for the homeless or disaster victims are good examples. At base, the intentions are worthy and those involved are seen to be doing good works. Many believe that such relatively small-scale projects shouldn't be scrutinised or evaluated because of their high moral content. There is little quibble with the good value inherent in stopping someone from taking a life in some, if not most, circumstances. We believe too little is expended on evaluating suicide prevention programmes. When public and private money is poured into such activities, there is a need to know how well or how badly the money and the energy are being expended, even if accountability brings unwanted or inconvenient results.

Evaluation in this context means to determine what preventions are working, and what are 'effective' means. (In Chap. 14 we discuss the role of review in organisations:

© Springer Nature Switzerland AG 2019   111
C. Tatz and S. Tatz, *The Sealed Box of Suicide*,
https://doi.org/10.1007/978-3-030-28159-5_9

whether decisions have been made well or badly, or need serious re-thinking.) Which jurisdictions or agencies are really preventing suicide, and how are they achieving this? Will a prevention or intervention that works in the affluent capital city of Canberra have efficacy on Inuit children living on Canada's remote Baffin Island? Does a programme that reduces suicide rates in unemployed older men in Eastern Europe have the same outcome when used on young women with eating disorders in California, and so on? Has 'zero suicide' been achieved anywhere, and if so, how?

We pause for a moment to outline the environment in which preventions are evaluated. First, suicide (as outlined in earlier chapters) is embedded in mental health and medicine, corralled along with other diseases and disorders. Those deemed suicidal may connect with suicide prevention agencies (such as crisis telephone services or NGOs) or find their way (voluntarily or not) to clinical and mental health treatments, often in acute settings. They are most often medicated, even physically restrained, before being discharged. Second, unlike other medical conditions, there is no clinical test, medical examination or device to identify who among us will suicide—unless individuals tell of their intention. Third, in the absence of a litmus test for suicide, the focus is on 'at-risk' groups who may or may not be potential suicides. (And we know that only a very small fraction of those labelled 'at-risk' do in fact make attempts or complete their exits.)

9.1 Suicide Prevention Agencies

Suicides are monitored at a national level in most countries; many have established national suicide prevention initiatives, including institutes, research centres and crisis services co-ordinating and delivering prevention activities. Across the globe, one finds agencies with names like Los Angeles Suicide Prevention Center, Suicide Prevention Australia, Lifeline, Crisis Line, American Association of Suicidology, National Suicide Prevention, the WHO European Network on Suicide Prevention, Centre de Prévention du Suicide, Beijing Suicide Research and Prevention Center, Suicide Ecoute, Alianţa Română de Prevenţie a Suicidului, Samaritans, R U OK? BeyondBlue, Stichting, SANE, Lifematters, and National Suicide Prevention Lifeline. These and hundreds (if not thousands) of other public and private organisations share commonalities: raising awareness of suicide through public education campaigns (especially in schools and among young people); reducing stigma; offering peer support; promoting early recognition and signs of suicide; championing evidence that suicide is preventable with the provision of appropriate mental health care and pharmacological treatment; focusing on issues like physical activity, diet, reducing alcohol and drug use; controlling the 'environment' (which includes means of suicide such as firearms, poisons et cetera) and restricting media coverage of suicide.

These prevention agencies undertake a range of interventions and mechanisms to stop suicides. Aside from important research, data collection and analysis, prevention agencies can deliver pioneering initiatives: preventing deaths on train and rail networks by changing lighting, music, signage and access, or in Guangzhou (China) where officials smeared butter over the climbable surfaces of the 1,000 foot long steel bridge known as a suicide 'hot spot'. Unlike traditional health preventions, suicide preventions adopt measures that are not legislative and are devoid of penalties or the types of 'stick and carrot' approaches proven in other prevention circumstances. Drink driving, for example, can be reduced through fines and tough penalties, while providing better access to other transport options and awareness of behaviour change (the designated driver, light beer and so on). The reductions in alcohol-related accidents and road trauma can be measured and world-wide comparisons evaluated.

Like road accidents, suicide rates differ within countries, regions, age cohorts, genders, religions, race and ethnicities; however, evaluation of prevention measures (outcomes) is far more fraught than measuring output. Suicide prevention analysis is much like the bloodletting regimen of yesteryear—it still comes under the rubric of 'observation'. Unlike the target of stopping road fatalities, the medical/mental health prevention approach cannot be properly evaluated because the factors underlying so many suicides are to be found in social contexts, situational conditions, economic and historical circumstances (not in evaluating the effect of building safer cars or better roads or penalising those who break the rules). Worth noting is the programme for the National Suicide Prevention Conference held in Melbourne in July 2019. Of the 140 or so presentations, not one was related to the contexts of suicide, to society, history, philosophy and sociology. Not surprising: the immediate socio-political context in Australia was and is a prime ministerial pronouncement that suicide is some kind of biblical or mediaeval curse, a health minister who wants five-year-olds sent to mental health clinics to be checked out (for potential suicidality), a governmental pledge for more psychology services and the major prevention agency wanting a federal ministerial portfolio to help solve the 'problem'.

9.2 What Is Being Evaluated?

Should the efficacy of suicide prevention programmes be troubling? Yes—because, unless we can dispassionately review the efforts of the last hundred years to prevent suicide, we will, like the war on drugs, continue to expend resources on measures and treatment that may only have limited impact; or more concerning, we will continue to use the same approaches, like the blood-letters, resistant to new paradigms and understandings.

Data are one component of evaluating prevention efficacy. As under-reported and variable as suicide data may be, at best it gives us indications and trends. World-wide, rates are not reducing, or not reducing systemically or uniformly, indicating at the very least that preventions are only partially achieving their aims. If statistics on suicide rates are the benchmark for preventionists' accomplishments, clearly the policies and programmes are meeting minimal success. Suicide rates have increased by 60% world-wide in the last 45 years, with international research indicating rising suicide rates within indigenous populations in the USA, Australia and New Zealand.[1] This may be a consequence of more accurate data. It could be that without prevention strategies the suicide rates would be much higher. Evaluations should answer this.

The activities of prevention agencies are easy to categorise; however, their achievements present as imprecise, even doubtful. Preventionists do things, lots of things. They create plans and strategies, they engage the public in high profile awareness-raising campaigns, they manage websites, build phone apps, produce reports and facts, host and attend endless conferences, forums, workshops and the all-important family and counsellor roundtable talks that can be effective. Suicide is now a priority of governments.

But the unanswered questions pile up. What are they preventing? All suicides, suicides of a defined age cohort or 'social class', suicides by a particular method or at a designated location? Are the preventions aimed at the young meant to be the same as those targeting middle-aged unemployed and isolated men? Are the strategies universal or selectively targeted? How do they account for variable economic, cultural, administrative and historical circumstances of suicides?

Suicide prevention, Knox et al. (2003) concluded, 'has not advanced significantly since Durkheim's work in the nineteenth century'. The impediment to progress lies in the tensions between the clinical and public health approaches to suicide. This applies to mental health more broadly; in Australia, psychosocial rehabilitation has been subjugated in favour of clinical care, with less than satisfactory outcomes for mental health consumers. Camus' belief that suicide was a truly philosophical problem has now been trumped by biomedicine and layers of entities promoting 'zero suicide' as achievable.

Widely disparate rates of suicide within and between countries more than suggests that evaluating ways to prevent suicide is inconsistent at best. Troubling, too, is the repeated assertion, the adamant assertion, that prevention and mental health always accompany each other. It is not conceivable that East Europeans experiencing the transformations from Stalinism to independence have more *mental illness* than Greeks, the latter undergoing a coincidental rise of self-deaths during their endless financial crises. Australians aren't ten times 'madder' than South Africans. Herein lies the dilemma of evaluating preventions—the medical approach studies individual behaviour and treats each case as if the suicidal person is divorced from community, culture, history, situation and circumstance. We agree with the view of Knox et al. (2003: 6) that 'suicide prevention remains rooted in a traditional but limited approach, that of clinical treatment of risk factors ... the results thus far are limited in their generalizability.'

---

[1] Suicide Statistics 2018. Befrienders Worldwide, citing WHO data. www.befrienders.org/suicide-statistics.

In their lengthy and well-researched paper on global suicide, WHO (2014) recognised that there 'is no single explanation of why people die by suicide'. In their *Prevention* chapter, WHO outlined the positives: 28 countries [to date] have national strategies committed to prevention; there are World Suicide Prevention Days and awareness/education campaigns. Medical professionals, self-help groups and crisis telephone lines exist in almost every country, along with risk assessments, interventions and support for the bereaved. And yet the WHO document, as comprehensive as it is, cannot tell us if these world-wide endeavours achieve their goals (WHO 2014: 6):

> A major design concern of any evaluation plan is the difficulty in attributing observed outcomes or impacts to the prevention strategy since many other factors could exert an influence on suicide rates and other indicators. For example, increased awareness and improved data may result in greater disclosure and more accurate information about suicides that would previously have been missed. This could result in apparently higher rates. Also, major changes such as economic crises can adversely affect population health and suicide by, for instance, reducing the financial capacity to respond to these issues. Consequently, understanding a strategy's context (history, organisation, and broader political and social setting) is essential and will improve how evaluations are conceived and conducted. There is a gap in the rigorous evaluation of promising suicide prevention strategies. While many new and innovative interventions have been noted and implemented internationally, they are yet to be evaluated. This is an issue particularly for low-income countries that may have learned valuable lessons in the implementation of suicide prevention that are lost due to a lack of data. The result is a bias towards interventions and recommendations from countries with an active academic sector.

WHO recognised the all-important external factors: that history, politics and social settings are essential criteria in evaluating suicide prevention strategies. But evaluations are based primarily on inputs and outputs: how many people saw an advertisement or poster, how many contacted a medical practitioner, how many called a telephone crisis line or how many participated in R U OK? Day (an Australian suicide awareness campaign based on 'starting a conversation'). Here is one example: in the Australian state of Victoria, the *Pause. Call. Be Heard.* campaign was designed to reduce deaths at Victorian train stations. It began in 2018 with billboards posted at selected railway stops. An evaluation by the University of Melbourne reported that 26% of randomly selected commuters had noticed these billboards, with 75% directly engaged with the messaging. We do not yet know the outcome; in Victoria, the suicide rate was hailed as falling in 2017—when three fewer persons took their lives than in the previous year.

What the prevention agencies do not (or cannot) account for is outcomes: to what extent did these specific interactions prevent suicide in the long-term? Did the person saved today not take his or her life later? Was it mental illness treatment or situation factors that prevented the suicide?

Experts in mental health prevention have had 'nearly a century of experience' Bertolote (2004) pointed out, with only 'a few but important lessons' to show. Bertolote's analysis of suicide preventions concluded with an important message:

'since suicide is affected by socio-cultural factors, there is no safe indication that what has worked somewhere will work elsewhere'. Althaus and Hegerl (2003) agreed that while 'one million people commit suicide world-wide every year and the need for suicide prevention is obvious … There is, however, but little evidence for the efficacy of suicide prevention activities'. They attributed this to 'methodological problems' in randomised controlled studies and insufficient sample sizes. They found that 'no single approach by itself seems to contribute to a substantial decline in the suicide rate'.

In their examination of suicide prevention strategies, Guo et al. (2003) also commented on the insufficient evidence to determine the effectiveness of prevention campaigns. Their research led them to conclude that, from the available evidence 'there is no single suicide prevention programme that appears to be effective in reducing suicide rates'. Looking specifically at the evaluation of suicide prevention programmes aimed at young people, the authors found 'insufficient evidence to support or not to support school-based suicide prevention programmes for adolescents'.

Another evaluation undertaken by researchers Dumesnil and Verger (2009) examined both public awareness and information campaigns that focused on depression and aimed to reduce suicide rates. Their specific attention was on well-known international programmes, such as *Like Minds, Like Mine* (New Zealand), *Changing Minds* (UK), *Choose Life* (Scotland) and world-wide Suicide Prevention Week programmes, along with Australian programmes, including 'mental health first aid', Victoria's Depression Awareness Research Project and Australia's leading mental health NGO, *beyondblue*. Reviewing 15 programmes across eight countries, they found only one evaluation was a randomised controlled trial; the others comprised public campaigns based on collective interventions with results unable to be allocated to individuals.

These researchers struggled to locate consistency or ways to compare prevention programmes and methods used to evaluate them. They found few reports pinpointed the 'epidemiologic, environmental, social and cultural context in which the programme was to be introduced', an essential component, they suggested, 'for determining what has been already done and what is needed by various population subgroups, for designing the programmes (objectives, target populations, methods, and means), and for collecting data for pre-post comparisons'. Their conclusion acknowledged that many and varied international awareness and prevention programmes targeting mental illness and depression have improved the general public's knowledge of suicide and depression and contributed 'at least moderately' to better social acceptance of depression and other mental illnesses; but 'it is difficult to establish whether these programmes help to increase care-seeking or to reduce suicidal behaviour' (Dumesnil and Verger 2009).

Scotland is held up as a model for emulation—it introduced funded and measurable public health strategies in public health fields, such as 'A Fairer Healthier Scotland 2017–22', an enviable strategy to reduce health inequalities and improve the Scottish population health, and a '10-year physical activity implementation plan'.

Their 'Suicide prevention action plan: every life matters' was launched in 2018 with the Minister for Mental Health, Clare Haughey, announcing, 'The Scottish Government believes that no death by suicide should be regarded as either acceptable or inevitable'. She reported that between 2002–2006 and 2013–2017 the rate of death by suicide in Scotland fell by 20%.[2] Yet in May 2018, a BBC news item quoted Professor Rory O'Connor, director of the Suicidal Behaviour Research Lab at Glasgow University:

> I've been studying suicide for the last 20-plus years and yes, our understanding of the complex set of factors have increased, but the stark reality is that we're no better than the flip of a coin at predicting who will kill themselves. If we focus in on men – between 70–75% of all suicides across the UK and Scotland are by men and we don't know enough about what it is about men, about the complex set of social, clinical and cultural factors and psychological factors that increase that risk.

It is worth highlighting that Scotland's suicide rates are more than two and a half times higher in the most deprived areas of that country. Alcohol misuse in Scotland has been identified as a factor, alongside poverty, inequity and, as Professor O'Connor highlighted, the complex set of factors that remain a sealed box, even to experts.

An analysis by Baker et al. (2018) of the European Alliance Against Depression programmes revealed mystifying variations: a 24% reduction in the number of suicidal acts (both suicide attempts and suicide deaths) and a significant reduction in the rate of suicide over a five-year period; contrasting with preliminary findings from ongoing evaluations of other European prevention programmes which reported no changes in rates in Germany and Hungary, and increases in Ireland. The conclusion, again, is for 'more research ... to understand the factors that moderate the effectiveness of this model and its sustainability in terms of reducing suicidal acts over the long term'. In their analyses of an American prevention programme called, rather optimistically, Zero Suicide, they found that even though more than 200 organisations are now implementing Zero Suicide and utilise their ten-step guide and Zero Suicide Toolkit, the outcomes are questionable. We too read with scepticism statistics boasting that the rate of suicide in the Henry Ford Health System of Michigan fell by 75%, when according to a recent Center for Disease Control study, the rate of suicide in Michigan had increased about 33%.

The 'important lessons' that José M. Bertolete said are derived from studying prevention include: a recognition that suicide prevention programmes cannot be transplanted, and that because one approach has worked for some people, or at some times, unless 'socio-cultural factors' are considered, they 'will probably yield frustrating results'.[3]

Countering the inability to prevent all suicide, and the questioning of prevention programmes, is the outcry for *more*—more funding, more investment in awareness-raising, more apps, more crisis lines, more starting of conversations, and most loudly,

---

[2]See: https://www.gov.scot/publications/scotlands-suicide-prevention-action-plan-life-matters/.
[3]http://www.ncbi.nlm.nih.gov/pmc/articles/PMC1414695/.

more funding for mental health services. The failure to reduce the rate of suicide is explained as a failure to invest *more* into existing preventions and interventions. We have attended suicide conferences where the failure is acknowledged—admissions that what we are doing isn't working—while paradoxically calling for more of the same. Preventions, we hear, are not to scale, are aimed too narrowly or not being rolled out nationally and internationally, they're missing the target audience; messages need refinements and refocussing; it is a problem of marketing and communications rather than the worthiness of suicide prevention campaigns.

9.3   Suicide Prevention in Australia

Our focus on Australia is intentional. OECD comparisons show Australia sits very comfortably relative to other OECD nations. The average disposable income and household net wealth are among the highest in the world; it has a low homicide rate and rates better than average across a range of health outcomes, including low birth weight, infant mortality, mortality from coronary heart disease, cancers and one of the lowest rates of tobacco smoking. The OECD *Better Life Index* showed that Australians were more satisfied with their lives than the OECD average, although as Rosenberg and Hickie (2018) cautioned, 'While international benchmarking can play an important role in fostering quality improvement, there are only limited mental health or social system performance data sources to utilise' (Rosenberg and Hickie 2018).

Another, darker country exists. Every day more than eight Australians die by suicide. In 2015, self-death accounted for 5.2% of all Aboriginal deaths compared to 1.8% for non-Aboriginal people. Lifeline Australia reported that there were approximately 65,300 suicide attempts each year in Australia.[4] The Australian Bureau of Statistics reported 3,128 people died from intentional self-harm (in 2017), a rise of 9.1% from 2016. A stark statistic, it equalled 2015 as the highest recorded preliminary rate of suicide in the past ten years. Intentional self-harm then ranked as the 13th leading cause of death, up from 15th position the year before.[5] The rise in suicides in Australia alarmed mental health and suicide prevention organisations. Despite their considerable labours, the number of people taking their own lives was increasing among some cohorts and not decreasing significantly in others.

The response was twofold: demands for more investment in mental health and a call for 'targets' that 'will focus the governments, funders and the community on

---

[4] www.lifeline.org.au/about-lifeline/lifeline-information/statistics-on-suicide-in-australia.

[5] www.abs.gov.au/ausstats/abs@.nsf/Lookup/by%20Subject/3303.0~2017~Main%20Features ~Intentional%20self-harm,%20key%20characteristics~3.

getting the numbers down and putting funding in all the right places'.[6] An Australian government spokesperson boldly stated: 'Australia does have a national target – zero suicides'. After a hundred years of prevention, the clarion call is for nebulous targets, as if proclaiming zero suicides will magically prevent the jumpers from jumping, the slashers from slashing and the hangers from hanging.

A national mental health and suicide prevention forum (Sydney, February 2019) ran under the tagline 'Reinforcing an integrated and person-centred care approach to improve mental health and advance "Zero Suicide"'. The speakers were predominately from the mental health field; the sessions focused on the individual, the outcome of the mythical 'zero suicides'. As with all such conferences, there is a substantial cost to attend the two-day event. How the poor, the alienated, the Aboriginal people from remote Australia, the socially isolated and lonely gain entry to understand their 'person-centred care' is not explained. As Australia's leading clinicians, academics and mental health professionals champion 'strategies for mental health reform to provide the best outcome for those experiencing mental illness and affected by suicide', others are less sanguine about existing preventions and evaluations.

At an Australian Labor Party National Health Policy Summit,[7] stakeholders said that not only was the current approach to suicide prevention failing, the actual suicide number was 'heading north, towards 4,000' (Mendoza 2017). Current suicide prevention strategies and initiatives were failing, and existing policy and funding policies were not going to realise any substantive changes.

A harsh but not unreasonable criticism of the Australian suicide and mental health sector is that it can be more focused on securing funding and raising awareness than providing critical analysis of the prevention framework or examining the individual, social and cultural factors accounting for suicide. Professor Ian Hickie, one of the country's most respected and outspoken clinicians, expressed his frustration with the proliferation of awareness campaigns for suicide prevention and mental health as different 'brands' competing for space in the media and for public funding, 'Australia is the most mental health literate country on earth by miles. The problem is not awareness. The problem is not being able to get a service'.[8] Others support Hickie's view, including Helen Christensen, chief scientist at the respected mental health research centre, Black Dog Institute (Christensen 2017):

> The past decade has seen significant sums of Australian government money dedicated to suicide prevention awareness activities. We've had websites, campaigns, summits and famous faces. Yet every year, we are seeing more people dying by suicide and more people making an attempt. It is trite and simplistic to think that simply raising awareness will fix the problem. Suicide is an extremely complex issue, involving myriad health, social, economic and personal factors that all need to be addressed before we can reduce our suicide rate.

---

[6] www.theguardian.com/australia-news/2018/sep/26/australias-rising-suicide-rate-sparks-calls-for-national-target-to-reduce-deaths.

[7] ALP National Health Summit, Parliament House, Canberra 3 March 2017.

[8] *Sun Herald Sunday* 30/4/2017: 12 Section: General News.

At a #StopSuicide Summit organised by Lifeline Australia, then CEO, Pete Shmigel, stated:

> Over the last decade, the rates of suicide and the net number of suicides in Australia has become an entrenched condition – we are facing a national suicide emergency. It is clear that what we're doing as a society right now is not working – and it needs to change. We know from Lifeline's 54 years of compassionate help-giving experience that there is more to suicide than mental illness.

As the main crisis telephone support service, Lifeline Australia deals directly with suicides and suicidality. Their own experience points to factors such as 'regional social and economic circumstances', including employment, financial status, social and income supports, the composition of households and family relationships. The interaction between these services and supports 'raises the prospect for more extensive service networks in suicide prevention plans than simply relying on contact with mental health services'.[9]

As some leading figures and organisations in the crisis/mental health/suicide field publicly challenge the prevailing norms and argue that suicide is not simply the inevitable consequence of mental illness, the current Australian government has reverted to the mediaeval language of breaking the 'curse' of suicide through the provision of more mental health services.

In the parallel universe of prevention, awareness-raising supplants evaluation. The *doing* is what counts. We have sighted the (confidential) strategy for World Suicide Prevention Day in Australia. It offers insights into how preventionists confuse outputs with outcomes. Their five-week campaign was designed to 'increase awareness and engagement' via a strategy based around a hashtag on social media, toolkits for hosting events, briefs for members of parliament, podcasts, 'digital assets' and a webinar. The key messages included an understanding 'that we all have a role in preventing suicide' and to promote two crisis lines if someone needs help. The language is motherhood: 'we need to work together to prevent suicide' and 'governments are funding and supporting the sector'. The public was asked to fundraise or host an event, 'start a conversation that matters' and to 'spread the word on social media'.

And how did they 'benchmark' the success of World Suicide Prevention Day? Certainly not by detailing how many people were prevented from self-harm or quantifying the impact on suicide rates. The measures of a successful prevention campaign were: increased monthly reach on Facebook by more than 3,000 and by Twitter by more than 40,000 impressions; achieving national and regional media coverage, hosting of 'a successful Webinar' and the creation of digital resources on a website. There is no evidence that any of these 'benchmarks' reduce suicide. To repeat, the rates went up. It was, and is, all about increasing funding and producing more outputs. No one has yet explained how money reduces suicide. Australia, or any nation, cannot buy its way out of suicide. T-shirt sales or sponsored walks around the country

---

[9]#StopSuicide Summit Briefing Pack. Lifeline Australia Summit, 1 May 2017, Sofitel Wentworth, Sydney.

achieve almost nothing but a feeling of doing something. Activities are not without importance to the bereaved and we applaud those well-meaning and dedicated people who staff the myriad mental health and suicide agencies and NGOs. But their efforts are largely ineffective without independent evaluations analysing whether all those tweets and Facebook posts that were 'liked' stop someone from suiciding. And if they did, did they stop them forever or was it a deflection or delay?

Fixating on outputs drives population health evaluations. In 2008, the Australian government launched the 'Measure Up' campaign, at a cost of tens of millions of dollars. Measure Up was designed to reduce the risks of chronic diseases such as heart disease, stroke and some cancers. The Australian Department of Health distributed 700,000 special tape measures as part of the campaign to raise appreciation of behavioural change and encourage Australians to increase their physical activity and adopt healthier eating habits. 'Measure Up' followed similar campaigns: 'Active Australia' (1997), 'Get Moving' (2006), 'Unplug and Play' (2008), 'Find Thirty' (2002) and 'Life, Be In It!' (1975). Evaluating 'Measure Up' showed, apparently, the money was well spent. The 'campaign achieved high unprompted (38%) and prompted (89%) awareness' boasted the evaluators. 'From pre- to post-campaign, knowledge and personal relevance of the link between waist circumference and chronic disease and waist measuring behaviour increased' they said, adding this incredible admission: 'although there were no significant changes in reported fruit and vegetable intake nor in physical activity'. Nonetheless, the evaluators concluded that 'Measure-Up' was 'successful at communicating the new campaign messages'.[10]

The 'Measure Up' campaign is cited for this reason: the multi-million dollar campaign was deemed successful for one reason only—the message was communicated. Never mind that more than half of Australian adults have a body weight that puts their health at risk; or that a few years post-'Measure Up' data revealed that 62% of Australian adults were overweight or obese, or that the proportion of adults who are obese/severely obese increased from 5% in 1995 to almost 10% in 2014. As Australia confronts a national obesity health crisis, the response by the current government is another multi-million dollar 'integrated national marketing and advertising campaign' called 'Move It'.

In Australia, prevention agencies similarly boast of their success. The reality we see questions this. Lifespan, an integrated suicide prevention programme run by the Black Dog Institute, vaunts its evidence-based approach to integrated suicide prevention. According to their published material, Lifespan uses a combination of nine strategies into one community-led approach, incorporating health, education, frontline services, business and the community. Their brochure asserts: 'Based on scientific modelling, LifeSpan is predicted to prevent 21% of suicide deaths, and 30% of suicide attempts'. At the time of writing, Lifespan programmes are being evaluated

---

[10]Evaluating the effectiveness of an Australian obesity mass-media campaign: how did the 'Measure-Up' campaign measure up in New South Wales?—PubMed—NCBI. www.ncbi.nlm.nih. gov. Health Educ Res. 2013 Dec; 28(6):1029–39. https://doi.org/10.1093/her/cyt084. Epub 2013 Aug 20. https://www.ncbi.nlm.nih.gov/pubmed/23962490.

in four regions (known as Primary Health Networks). Amid rising rates in Australia, this startling claim of 21% reduction is surely the breakthrough in prevention. But preliminary evaluations mirror other findings—they simply cannot say for certain if their methods are working. Despite the ambitious claims one in five suicides can be reduced, this is what the evaluation from the Lifespan and Black Dog Institute reported (Baker et al. 2018):

> LifeSpan … await[s] comprehensive evaluation. Until then, it may be premature to draw conclusions on the overall effectiveness of multi-component systems approaches to suicide prevention. In particular, important questions remain regarding the feasibility and effectiveness of large-scale implementation. Further work on a larger scale is required to provide more evidence.

Evaluation and accountability are essential, not just to hold government and NGOs to justify their funding and programme deliverability; accountability allows suicide researchers to analyse if the methods and approaches to prevention are working. And if not, to question, as we are doing here, alternative approaches.

Evaluations of suicide prevention programmes in Australia and overseas do produce evidence. Strategies to reduce death by pesticides or drowning, or among particular cohorts, have produced short-term impacts but long-term trends, and outside factors (social upheaval, global financial crises and growing inequities) render most evaluations inconclusive. In the end, suicide prevention is both a 'product' and a service and in whatever way one looks at the activities, some questions need answers. Does it work, and for whom? The preventionists and/or the 'clients', 'patients', the recipients? Did the client want the service and, if still alive, is there any indication of gratitude or some other emotion? Are those prevented still alive a year later, five or ten years on? While the strictest privacy would or should pervade these actions, anonymous numbers can still be meaningful. How many were saved in the past year? By what means? Was there follow up? Is there ongoing follow up? Are there what doctors would call after-care or on-going post-discharge monitoring? Do these agencies keep records of named 'clients' so that evidence of prevention can be elicited? Are there meetings in the way that Alcoholics Anonymous operates? Is there 'rehab', that is, ongoing therapies that seek to avoid relapses? Are there programmes that seek to provide employment for those who sought a way out of financial stringency? Housing for those who were homeless? Collegiality for those who were alone? Reconnections for those who were disconnected? Do we, or the preventionists, have any idea of how many were contacted initially, dissuaded from suicide initially and then took their lives?

The answers vary. Yes to some, in part or no to others. It depends on who you are: your age, gender, race, ethnicity, language skills and health literacy; where you live, whether you can afford private health and support services. And financial wherewithal and income, relationships and connections, drug and alcohol use. The list goes on.

Given that suicide rates generally are increasing, what does appraisal of preventionism tell us, and what does it say to those engaged in that domain? The billions of dollars poured into research and treatment in the 'war on cancer' has produced some positive results in a handful of that disease's forms. The war on drugs is futile, yet the slowish movements to decriminalise some drugs begin to make some sense. The 'war on suicide', without the investments that cancer and illicit drugs receive, cannot be 'won' in the sense of 'zero suicide' targets. But suicide can be alleviated, mitigated, deflected in some cases—but only when we know the contexts of rescue programmes and the reliability of the approaches used. In short, without more disciplined, more carefully constructed evaluation processes, preventionism can't prevent.

References

Althaus, D., & Hegerl, U. (2003). The evaluation of suicide prevention activities: State of the art. *The World Journal of Biological Psychiatry, 4*(4), 156–165.

Baker, S. T. E., Nicholas, J., Shand, F., Green, R., & Christensen, H. (2018). A comparison of multi-component systems approaches to suicide prevention. *Australasian Psychiatry, 26*(2), 128–131. Article first published online: November 21, 2017; Issue published April 1 https://journals.sagepub.com/doi/full/10.1177/1039856217743888.

Bertolote, J. M. (2004, October). Suicide prevention: At what level does it work? *World Psychiatry* (3). https://www.ncbi.nlm.nih.gov/pmc/articles/PMC1414695/.

Christensen, H. (2017, May 3). Raising awareness around suicide isn't enough to fix the problem. *Huffington Post*.

Dumesnil, H., & Verger, P. (2009). Public awareness campaigns about depression and suicide: A review. http://ps.psychiatryonline.org/doi/full/10.1176/ps.2009.60.9.1203.

Guo, B., Scott, A., & Bowker, S. (2003). Prevention strategies: Evidence from systematic reviews. Alberta Heritage Foundation for Medical Research, 19. www.researchgate.net/publication/265074097_Suicide_Prevention_Strategies_Evidenefrom.

Knox, K. L., Conwell, Y., & Caine, E. (2003). If suicide is a public heath problem, what are we doing to prevent it? *American Journal of Public Health, 94*(1), 37–45.

Mendoza, J. (2017). CEO of ConNetica, at ALP national Health Summit (Suicide and Mental Health section), March 3.

Rosenberg, S., & Hickie, I. (2018). No gold medals: Assessing Australia's international mental health performance. *Australasian Psychiatry, 27*(1), 36–40, February 2019. https://doi.org/10.1177/1039856218804335. Epub October 8, 2018.

WHO. (2014). Preventing suicide: A global imperative. WHO Library Cataloguing-in-Publication Data. World Health Organization. ISBN 978-92-4-156477-9 (NLM classification: HV 6545) © World Health Organisation.

Chapter 10
The Assisters

I will give no deadly medicine to any one if asked nor suggest
any such counsel...

—The Hippocratic Oath

Voluntary euthanasia occurs only when to the best of medical
knowledge a person is suffering from an incurable and painful
or extremely distressing condition. In these circumstances one
cannot say that to choose to die quickly is obviously irrational.

—Peter Singer [Australian moral philosopher]

Abstract A history of euthanasia; categories of euthanasia; death as kindness is not a suicide; the medical profession and euthanasia; opposition to physician-assisted death; legal assisted dying across the world; Victoria's euthanasia laws; anomalies in who may request assisted death; Exit International.

Keywords Euthanasia · Assisted dying · Physician-assisted suicide

In Sydney, we know half a dozen ageing couples who have taken Mexican vacations—not for any love of chocolate-cooked food or the tacos but because that is the source of Nembutal, a lethal barbiturate promoted by euthanasia movements as the 'peaceful pill', the gentle way out. The degree of premeditation, the rational afterthought and the cost factor make this a remarkable behaviour. There is a total absence of impulsivity. This is neither a hallucinatory moment nor 'a senior's moment'. Nor is this an outcome of mental illness, a condition that is unlikely to be consistent with the high degree of planning and preparation. Many Nembutal buyers belong to Dying with Dignity groups: that takes the meaning of *intent*, sentient intent, to a new level.

© Springer Nature Switzerland AG 2019
C. Tatz and S. Tatz, *The Sealed Box of Suicide*,
https://doi.org/10.1007/978-3-030-28159-5_10

10.1   Euthanasia

Εὐθανασία is a Greek word; 'eu' means 'goodly' or 'well' and 'thanatos' is 'death', hence a 'good death'. The English translation is euthanasia, a word representing the process of intentionally terminating a person's life in order to reduce their pain and suffering.

The *good* death is the converse of *bad* suicide. The former connotes mercy-killing, an understandable desire to end suffering, to die with dignity, and clearly not a stigmatised self-harm. Euthanasia is couched in the language and imagery of ending suffering in a humane and decent way; respectfully, at peace. Euthanasia brings to mind another Greek concept, *autonomy*, derived from *auto* meaning 'self' and *nomos* which means 'custom' or 'law'. Autonomy describes people able to make choices of their own free will, or make decisions independently from authority figures. For many, it remains sinful, a blasphemy in which the individual is asserting their will over or against that of God, the divine who alone dispenses life.

Euthanasia is beset by moral and ethical questions: when is it legally acceptable to take your own life, or assist another to end theirs? What circumstances justify the termination of life? How does the state differentiate morally between letting a person die and actively hastening their death? Who decides on the right to die? What is the difference between euthanasia and suicide?

Euthanasia and suicide are perceived as distinct, separate and disconnected. Suicide is unexpected: it jars and shocks. It is unexpected, even when signs of intent are evident. No leaping from buildings or hanging from ropes, euthanasia conjures images of an elderly person, rent by untreatable disease and abject pain, allowed to die serenely. There are moral ambiguities or 'grey areas' about suicide. One cannot be 'pro-suicide' in the way pro-euthanasia is accepted. Planning for euthanasia is rational, premeditated. Neurological dysfunctions and genetic aberrations require no investigation. Ending suffering and alleviating terminal pain inhabit discourse and debate far removed from suicide prevention and mental illness.

Debates on euthanasia—in courts of law, legislatures, medical associations and public conversations—are grounded in the complexities of mental capacity, what constitutes 'life', how self-determination and autonomy are assessed, religious doctrine, individual rights and the role of the medical profession in assisted dying. Suffering and pain are neither dismissed nor rejected in euthanasia dialogues; the question is whether a person has the right to end life. Euthanasia, even to those who oppose it, is understood. The reality of pain is not disputed. The ultra-religious may offer reasons, the hopeful may believe in magic cures, the palliative care specialists may claim they can palliate pain, but understanding suffering is never questioned.

Most people 'get' euthanasia. We understand it from a personal perspective because we can appreciate untreatable pain. For the living, family and friends, euthanasia relieves their suffering and pain. Mercy-killing, as it is often called, or was once the popular term, is accepted—in some jurisdictions legally, in others tacitly. If one articulates the desire to end one's life—through voluntary euthanasia, or via an Advance Directive[1]—you are not considered in need of medication or psychiatric care. Substitute euthanasia for suicide and the same expression to cease living is transformed into a condition or disease that must be prevented at all costs.

There are important distinctions in this manner of death: voluntary euthanasia, non-voluntary, involuntary and active or passive euthanasia. We will not be addressing the realities of state murder, as in the Nazi 'cleansing' policy of *Lebensunwerten Lebens* (sanctioning the taking of life unworthy of life). (The booklet giving rise to that notion came from jurist Karl Binding and psychiatrist Alfred Hoche. The consequent exercise in biopower, the T4 programme, ran from 1933 until three weeks *after* World War II ended and operated under the banner of the German Red Cross.) We concentrate here on assisted dying, a voluntary suicide by a person requesting help in ending intolerable living.

10.2 Death as Kindness

The Prince of Denmark, in Shakespeare's *Hamlet* (Act III, Scene I), questioned whether to live or die ('to be or not to be'). Death, pondered the melancholic Hamlet: 'To sleep: perchance to dream: ay, there's the rub; For in that sleep of death what dreams may come, When we have shuffled off this mortal coil'. It is peaceful death Hamlet contemplated, a chance to dream. Indeed, euthanasia today is achieved through sedative medications that offer a Shakespearean passing; dying painlessly as an act of kindness.

Another playwright, Brian Clarke, in 1972 penned *Whose Life Is It Anyway* (later released as a motion picture in 1981); it also brought euthanasia to mainstream audiences. Clarke's play centred on Ken Harrison, a happy, active sculptor rendered paraplegic following a motor accident. Told he would never recover, Harrison was incapable of creativity, sex or any 'normal' life; his existence was sustained through hospital technology. When his wish to end his life (by being discharged from the hospital) was denied, Harrison sought legal redress, petitioning the court to allow him the right to choose to die.

Initially, the hospital doctors decided to commit Harrison on the grounds he was suicidal and mentally unwell, for no person of right mind chooses to terminate a life. The 'shrinks' were at odds—was this patient intelligent, sane, rational, one who desired to die at home with dignity, or a person of unsound mind? Challenging his doctors and psychiatrists, Harrison argued that patients could, and should, have

---

[1]An advance care directive (Advance Directive), also known as a 'living will', refers to a legal document that provides directives, with legally binding instructions about future medical treatment, end-of-life care and preferences for medical treatment.

autonomy over medical decisions. His wish to be discharged and die a dignified death at home was portrayed as a perfectly normal reaction to his situation. 'I do not want to die', Harrison said at one point, 'I am dead already'. His circumstances didn't constitute a life: he was helpless, cruelly deprived of any enjoyment of life; an artist trapped in a body that couldn't create; a sharp, witty and observant mind deteriorating in a body unable to function at even the most basic level; a sexually active man reduced to impotent flirting with his nurse.

Harrison was tortured by his imagination. What could have been was no longer possible. He pleaded: 'my mind, which had been my most precious possession, has become my enemy and it tortures me. It tortures me with thoughts of what might have been, and what might be to come and I can feel my mind, very slowly, breaking up'. The dramatic denouement is the judge's verdict. Faced with judging whether Harrison had a moral, ethical and legal right to choose to die, the judge granted Harrison's wish. Audiences were intellectually and emotionally sated. The play/movie delivered sensitive and articulate dialogue about the right to die. The reality of euthanasia is often far removed from such staged scenarios.

10.3   Forms of Euthanasia

As with suicide, euthanasia has differing classifications: active, passive, voluntary, involuntary, assisted and physician-assisted.

Active euthanasia describes situations where an outside agent or force has caused a death, such as by lethal injection or other means of administering lethal medications or drugs that hasten death. Active is clearly distinct from passive; it is an action that deliberately and directly *causes* a patient's death. For some, perhaps many, *active* euthanasia is murder.

Passive euthanasia describes treatments or forms of life support that are removed or denied. *Whose Life Is It Anyway?* was about the passive category. The Harrison character was not killed, but he could not live for long without the aid of medical technology, his discharge would ensure death. Passive euthanasia most commonly occurs when life-support machines are switched off, feeding tubes disconnected or life-extending medications are withdrawn. So we have euthanasia by commission and by omission. Actions, wrote euthanasia expert Dr. Richard Huxtable, are thought to be 'worse than omissions, even if omissions have the same effect as the actions' (Huxtable 2013: 131). The disconnecting of life-supporting machinery is seen—morally, ethically?—as less worse than delivering a lethal injection. Death is graded. A suicide by overdose is somehow less confronting than the jumper from an office building. Gently turning off a switch is, to many, a world removed from a syringe full of lethal chemicals.

Voluntary euthanasia involves a distinct request to terminate one's life made by a person considered capable and competent in making such a decision. Competence is the keyword here, as is the capacity of the requestor and their ability to communicate their intent.

Involuntary euthanasia describes death where a patient is not fully competent and capable of making life or death decisions, such as being comatose or rendered incapable of making a rational decision.

Assisted suicide is used to describe a situation where a person, having made the decision to end their life, requires another person or persons to assist them.

Physician-assisted euthanasia involves a medical practitioner ending a person's life, most commonly through medication. Assisted suicide occurs when a doctor provides the means for a person to end a life, such as prescribing medication that can be taken in lethal doses but does not administer it themselves.

For the medical profession, the distinction between *killing* and *letting die* is critical.

10.4 Doctors and Euthanasia

Physician-assisted suicide divides medical associations and medical practitioners. Medical associations oppose any involvement of doctors in hastening death. The World Mental Health Association's Declaration on Euthanasia[2] adopted by the 38th World Medical Assembly in October 1987 (and then reaffirmed by the 170th WMA Council Session in France in May 2005) stated:

> Euthanasia, that is, the act of deliberately ending the life of a patient, even at the patient's own request or at the request of close relatives, is unethical. This does not prevent the physician from respecting the desire of a patient to allow the natural process of death to follow its course in the terminal phase of sickness.

The WMA Statement on Physician-Assisted Suicide was similar:

> Physician-assisted suicide, like euthanasia, is unethical and must be condemned by the medical profession. Where the assistance of the physician is intentionally and deliberately directed at enabling an individual to end his or her own life, the physician acts unethically. However, the right to decline medical treatment is a basic right of the patient and the physician does not act unethically even if respecting such a wish results in the death of the patient.

Even though it recognises that euthanasia is legalised in some countries, the WMA 'strongly encourages all national medical associations and physicians to refrain from

---

[2]See: https://www.wma.net/policies-post/wma-declaration-on-euthanasia/.

participating in euthanasia, even if national law allows it or decriminalizes it under certain conditions'.

The Australian Medical Association (AMA, or AuMA as it is known internationally) best describes the nuanced position of the right to let a patient die and the role of doctors assisting in death. Medical practitioners, the AuMA wrote in its 2016 Position Statement *Euthanasia and Physician Assisted Suicide*,[3] have 'an ethical duty to care for dying patients so that death is allowed to occur in comfort and with dignity'. Doctors have a responsibility to initiate and provide good quality end-of-life care and should strive to make sure their patients who are dying are free from pain and suffering. They must also endeavour 'to uphold the patient's values, preferences and goals of care'. For the AuMA, not initiating life-prolonging measures, not continuing life-prolonging measures, or not administering treatments that may have a secondary consequence of hastening death, does not constitute euthanasia. It is 'interventions that have as their primary intention the ending of a person's life' that the AuMA— and every other medical association—opposes. Importantly, the Australian Medical Association recognised 'there are divergent views within the medical profession and the broader community in relation to euthanasia and physician assisted suicide'; and the ultimate decisions on the legality of euthanasia and physician-assisted suicide rests with governments and not with individuals.

The American Medical Association is hardly subtle in its opposition to euthanasia. They do acknowledge the desire to end suffering and painful illness as *understandable*, however, 'permitting physicians to engage in euthanasia would ultimately cause more harm than good'. For the USA's peak medical body, euthanasia 'is fundamentally incompatible with the physician's role as healer, would be difficult or impossible to control and would pose serious societal risks. Euthanasia could readily be extended to incompetent patients and other vulnerable populations'.[4]

Media coverage of the AMA House of Delegates debate on physician-assisted euthanasia oftentimes referred to polling indicating overwhelming public support for euthanasia. Australian polling indicates similar public support. The public may (and we accepted that polling is subject to variances and is at best an indication of trends and general position) support voluntary euthanasia, however the medical profession sees its role as keeping patients alive, even against their wishes. Through the marvels of modern medical science, doctors can keep patients breathing; they may be in agony, they may suffer physically and mentally, they may wish to end their lives, but without legislation, doctors have the right to make life and death decisions, not the individuals.

Physicians hold up the Hippocratic Oath as their commandment not to assist in death. Written almost 2500 years ago, allegedly by the Greek physician called Hippocrates of Kos, the origins of the Oath are curious. The Oath originally called on physicians to swear by 'Apollo, by Asclepius, by Hygieia, by Panacea, and by all

---

[3] See: https://ama.com.au/media/euthanasia-and-physician-assisted-suicide.

[4] See: https://www.ama-assn.org/delivering-care/ethics/euthanasia.

the gods and goddesses, making them my witnesses, that I will carry out, according to my ability and judgment, this oath and this indenture'. The original Oath did not include the much-quoted phrase 'first do no harm'. That dictum arrived centuries later when the Hippocratic Oath was translated and used as a recital by graduating doctors. In the 1960s, a secular version was created removing the need for gods to witness the passage of medical students.

It is to the Oath that physicians turn when opposing euthanasia. For these medicos, *do no harm* means not assisting a patient to end their life, irrespective of their autonomy, wishes, advance directives, patient-centred care, untreatable pain or the potential for suicide. Their creed is the opposite of the retail/hospitality mantra of 'the customer is always right'. To end one's life, for whatever reasons, can never be 'right' for the medical profession.

The modern interpretation of any text written thousands of years ago is certainly questionable. The Hippocratic Oath, for example, prohibited abortion ('I will not give a woman a pessary to cause an abortion'), surgery ('I will not use the knife, even upon those suffering from stones') and mandatory reporting to authorities ('Whatever I see or hear in the lives of my patients, whether in connection with my professional practice or not, which ought not to be spoken of outside, I will keep secret, as considering all such things to be private'). Like the Bible, doctors opposing physician-assisted suicide pick and choose parts of the Hippocratic Oath.

Leon Kass from the University of Chicago penned an article titled 'Neither for Love nor Money: Why Doctors Must Not Kill' (1989). There are myriad articles and papers of similar bent, but this one stands out as Kass is explicit in positioning medicine as a moral profession, where the dignity and mysterious power of human life itself is inspirational:

> The deaths we most admire are those of people who, knowing that they are dying, face the fact frontally and act accordingly: they set their affairs in order, they arrange what could be final meetings with their loved ones, and yet, with strength of soul and a small reservoir of hope, they continue to live and work and love as much as they can for as long as they can. Because such conclusions of life require courage, they call for our encouragement—and for the many small speeches and deeds that shore up the human spirit against despair and defeat.

For this doctor, and we suspect others with similar views, courage and hope take precedence over the rational mind. A certain God-like aura accompanies pronouncements of this ilk. Here, we witness physicians discovering mysteries, hope and purity where their patients (and families) experience abject pain, torture, torment and slow and agonising death.

Keith Macdonald's *The Sociology of the Professions* (1995) is illuminating on the matter of the professions, their status, power and knowledge. Strangely, he didn't talk about morality and the professions but has an interesting pair of chapters, one on the caring professions and another on the uncaring ones. Solicitors and accountants he declared uncaring. Doctors and nurses were implicitly in the former category. If morality is the issue, or an issue, one has to question the conceit that what medical people do is *always* in the best interests of the patient. It is obvious from the debates surrounding assisted dying that a great many physicians appear to be more concerned with societal morality, governmental morality, than patient considerations. When a person is terminally ill, in utter torment, and medicine knows that there is no more to be done, whose morality is being kept intact by prolonging such a 'life'?

This is not the place for a full discussion of medical behaviour across the ages. But the high moral ground of never taking a life but always preserving one rings all too hollow in history. The major roles played by physicians in the Armenian and Jewish genocides have been fully documented, as has the part played by Russian psychiatrists in the Soviet Union days, the role of doctors in the Bosnian rape centres in the 1990s and so on. Since 1977 in America, some 919 executions have taken place by lethal injection. Doctors accept a fee for delivering that service. However much immunity they may have for a state-sanctioned judicial killing, taking a healthy life is what they are doing.

10.5   Psychological Suffering and Euthanasia

To paraphrase Albert Camus, there is another serious philosophical problem—why people living with pain and suffering of other dimensions—mental, emotional, psychological, situational—must be prevented from taking their lives, yet those with physical pain can (legally or due to the non-enforcement of the law by authorities), through their own agency, or with assistance, be aided to shuffle from this mortal coil before 'their time has come'? Is not mental pain, psychological suffering and the desire to terminate one's life to prevent days, weeks, months or years of agony not a reason for voluntary euthanasia? Why is terminal illness an acceptable reason to die with dignity, but not terminal despair, loneliness, trauma, disability or mental illness?

At this time of writing (mid-2019), euthanasia is legally practised in six states in the USA (Hawaii, Washington, Oregon, Colorado, Vermont, California, with Montana allowing physician-assisted suicide via court rulings). Canada passed medically assisted dying laws in 2016, and the Australian state of Victoria enacted a statute in 2017. In a rapidly changing political-legal environment, active assisted dying is currently legal in the Netherlands, Belgium and Luxembourg. Germany, Switzerland, Austria and Finland permit physician-assisted death under specific circumstances. England, Spain, Sweden, Italy, Hungary and Norway permit passive euthanasia under strict circumstances. Each of these nations has enacted different or differing legislative and legal regulations, with only three countries that we know of (Belgium, Luxembourg and the Netherlands) not restricting euthanasia to just physical suffering.

Euthanasia on the grounds of psychological suffering is rarely accepted. Research was undertaken by Verhofstadt et al. (2017) into suffering experienced by psychiatric patients requesting euthanasia. We cite this particular study as it provides a comprehensive outline of mental illness and euthanasia. As noted above, in Belgium, Luxembourg and The Netherlands, patients can request euthanasia for both untreatable and unbearable suffering. Belgium and Luxembourg are at present the only nations with legislation specifying that both physical and/or psychological suffering are legitimate reasons for requesting euthanasia. Five 'domains' of 'unbearable suffering' were identified: medically related suffering, intrapersonal and interpersonal suffering, societal suffering related to one's place and interactions and existential suffering (Verhofstadt et al. 2017). The latter two interests us.

'Unbearable suffering', these research authors pointed out, is only known by the patient. The relationship between physical suffering (terminal illnesses, untreatable pain) and mental distress is not easily distinguishable in the context of seeking voluntary euthanasia. How does one gauge the psychological suffering of a terminally ill patient navigating the medico-legal bureaucracy of assisted dying processes? Verhofstadt and her colleagues reported that financial pressures (including concerns about medical expenses), difficulties in coping with the 'rat race', inability to adjust, feelings of burdening society, loneliness and isolation were factors in societal suffering linked to requests for euthanasia. In the existential category, a fear of loss of quality of life, loss of control (autonomy), being treated as a puppet (or guinea pig) by physicians, detachment from their bodies and the futility of continuing medical care were reported (Verhofstadt 2017).

10.6 Euthanasia in Victoria (Australia)

In June 2016, the Parliament of Victoria, an Australian state with a population of 6.4 million, held an inquiry into voluntary euthanasia. We cite the government's *Inquiry into End of Life Choices*[5] as it proved to be a wide-ranging and fascinating insight into the arguments and positions adopted by the pro- and anti-euthanasia groups in what is considered a progressive state in one of the richest and most advanced nations in the world.

Victoria's parliament, after lengthy and at times acrimonious debate, passed legislation sanctioning euthanasia from 2019 under certain conditions. The Inquiry provided a platform for all and sundry to air their views, including whether psychological suffering and mental illness were grounds for an application for euthanasia. Some interesting background information emerged from the extensive public deliberation. Suicide was decriminalised in Victoria in 1967, however, up to five years

---

[5]The full report (*Inquiry into End of Life Choices*) and transcripts of hearings, which are cited, can be found at: https://www.parliament.vic.gov.au/lsic/inquiries/article/2611.

in jail potentially awaits anyone who incites a person to take his or her own life. To date, no person has been prosecuted for this offence. The Committee Inquiry heard that the laws do not align with the community's views that leniency is always offered in cases of assisted dying, a situation mirrored in other Australian jurisdictions and internationally. Punishment is deemed unnecessary and unwarranted, offenders are unlikely to ever re-offend, and rehabilitation is pointless. Despite evidence of individuals assisting in another's death, upholding the black letter of the law served no public purpose. Neither the police nor prosecuting authorities pursue suspected cases of doctors or others assisting in dying.

The arguments against euthanasia are by now universal. Euthanasia evokes Nazi Germany. The vulnerable, frail and disabled will be put down, or believing they are burdensome, will seek early death. It is a slippery slope—what may begin as a restricted practice degenerates into the wholesale killing of elderly and vulnerable people. The mentally ill and those with suicidal intent will find ways to use legislation to kill themselves. Those close to death are often in a coma or sedated into semiconsciousness, they are not experiencing pain and suffering. Palliative care meets the needs of dying patients. We have addressed the physicians' position earlier.

Religious opposition to euthanasia is well known. Christianity and Judaism have an uncompromising view that the body belongs to God and that only the Deity can give and take life. Involuntary euthanasia is, of course, considered beyond the pale. At Australian parliamentary inquiries into euthanasia, Christian and Jewish representatives railed against any interference in the life cycle. God giveth and God taketh, although they are less vocal about God's policy on heart transplants, blood transfusions and artificial insemination. The sanctity of life is His (always in the masculine gender) and His alone.

Buddhism is based on a set of principles rather than a code of morality. The essence is to do no harm, and so assisted dying would probably be considered harm. Orthodox Judaism holds that taking a life even in the immediacy of death is unlawful killing (Akiva Tatz 2010: 153).

But attitudes towards voluntary assisted dying are now seen to be softening in the face of 'exceptional psychological stress' or 'mental ill health'. The same is happening with suicide. For example, a Catholic priest officiating at a teenager's funeral in America on December 2018 made a speech in which he doubted the boy would enter heaven because he took his life. The outraged family complained, and the priest was stood down (BBC News, 16.12.2018). The deceased 'had issues', presumably of the disordered kind.

Andrew Denton, a popular Australian TV and radio personality and author, led a public campaign for legislated euthanasia. At the above-mentioned Victoria Inquiry, Denton delivered persuasive testimony, relating examples gleaned from examining euthanasia in Belgium where 'initially I found it (mental suffering) extremely confronting, because I did not understand then what I understand now, which is that psychiatric suffering—long-term what they call therapy-resistant psychiatric pain—can be equal to or in excess of any known physical pain'.[6]

Denton told the story of Pierre, whose daughter first exhibited severe mental illness in her teens. Diagnosed with bulimia, she began to cut and burn herself. Committed to an institution, the young woman was assessed by 'psychiatrist after psychiatrist' yet she continued to self-harm and attempted suicide several times. Pierre took his daughter to Belgian doctors, pleading to allow her to be euthanased. They refused. Denton described the consequence: 'At the age of 31, having suffered like this for 14 years, somehow or other in a lockup psychiatric institution, (the daughter) managed to cut her own throat and finally kill herself'. As Denton acknowledged, it is a challenging issue for psychiatrists to recommend a patient be allowed to die. Suicide, which is an alternative, is even more challenging. Yet only a very small percentage of people experiencing existential or psychological distress seek euthanasia. The request for euthanasia is often the 'alarm bell' initiating appropriate support and treatment.

Three Victorian coroners gave insightful testimony in relation to euthanasia and suicide (English et al. 2015). The first case they raised was a 59-year-old man, in a loving marriage of 38 years, with no history of mental illness, yet bearing the diagnosis of metastatic cancer. After 22 cycles of treatment, his prognosis remained dire. Admitted to hospital, the patient expressed his desire to go home to die, telling his family he would suicide rather than die in a hospital bed after a period of suffering. It is not clear how he left the hospital but the patient was later found hanging from a bridge with a suicide note indicating his intentions. In another case, an 82-year-old woman, living alone, became depressed as her physical health deteriorated. She was unable to read her beloved books, which were said to be the most important part of her life. Her doctors described her as (in Denton's words) 'lonely, isolated, frustrated, impatient'. She told her children many times of her desire to die. Later, this 82-year-old woman cut herself with a serrated knife and died by loss of blood.

It would be stories like these—suicides by people who begged to end their life with dignity and through their own choice—that persuaded the Victorian parliament to (narrowly) pass assisted dying legislation. The *Voluntary Assisted Dying Act* limits voluntary assisted dying (VAD) to people over 18 years of age who are terminally ill and who fulfil very strict criteria in relation to experiencing unrelievable physical suffering. They must possess sufficient decision-making capabilities and be in the last six months of life (those with neurodegenerative disease must be in the last 12 months of life). The Act specifically states: 'A person is not eligible for access to voluntary assisted dying only because the person is diagnosed with a mental illness, within the meaning of the *Mental Health Act 2014*'.

If not an example of discrimination this certainly is an example of the ongoing stigma associated with mental illness; those with mental illness (often unable to

---

[6]Andrew Denton's testimony can be found at Inquiry into End of Life Choices and transcripts of hearings: https://www.parliament.vic.gov.au/lsic/inquiries/article/2611.

access proper mental health care) are not allowed the right to die with dignity; that right is prescribed only for the physically ill.

For those who wish to discontinue living yet are deemed ineligible, or who live in other Australian jurisdictions, suicide or travelling overseas to facilities that end life remain the only options.

10.7   Exit International

Philip Nitschke is a former physician and founder of the pro-euthanasia group Exit International. In 1996, Dr. Nitschke gained world-wide attention when he became the first physician to administer a legal—and lethal—injection to a patient wanting voluntary euthanasia. Nitschke performed this under the *Rights of the Terminally Ill Act 1995* of the Northern Territory (NT).

Dr. Nitschke is now Mr. Nitschke. His medical registration was suspended by the Australian Medical Board in July 2014 and although the NT Supreme Court overruled this decision, he subsequently burned his medical registration certificate. He is, along with American pathologist Jack Kevorkian, one of the most recognised advocates of euthanasia. The nickname 'Dr. Death' accompanies media coverage on both Nitschke and Kevorkian.

Nitschke's battle with Australian authorities ignited a complex constitutional fight that pitted the Commonwealth government against a designated jurisdiction whose elected government had granted individuals the right to choose to end their life once specific conditions had been satisfied. Australia has two territories—the Northern Territory (NT), a vast area (1.42 million km^2) known as the 'outback' with a population of only 250,000; and the Australian Capital Territory (ACT), a small region (2,358 km^2) with about 420,000 residents. As Territories (and not States), the Australian Constitution has a loophole which permits the Commonwealth (federal) government to make laws governing the Territories. After the conservative Chief Minister of the NT, Marshall Perron, successfully introduced voluntary euthanasia legislation—allowing Dr. Nitschke to perform four end-of-life procedures—a right-wing federal conservative member, Kevin Andrews MP, used this rarely known loophole to quash the rights of Territorians to access voluntary euthanasia. The 'Kevin Andrews Bill' as it became known rendered it illegal for the Northern Territory government to make laws allowing euthanasia.

Before the Commonwealth overrode the NT statute, a patient with end-stage prostate cancer was given lethal drugs from what was dubbed a 'death machine'—a computer-operated device that released lethal drugs once the patient had activated the equipment. The machinations of the Australian government are significant. Until Victoria passed euthanasia laws we saw unheralded and heavy-handed use of government power to prohibit the right to choose to die. Nitschke turned his expertise to found Exit International. On their website, Exit International reminds us that 'Dying is not a medical process. As such, the dying process does not always (or ever) need to involve the medical profession'.[7] The medical profession would beg to differ.

Today, Switzerland is the destination for Australians and others opting for an end-of-life choice. Exit International says there is a lengthy and extensive process to access their 'service', and it is not cheap—around US$7,500 (airfares not included). We are unable to find accurate information on how many people have travelled overseas for the procedure. For those unable to travel, the dark web contains sites offering advice on suicide and euthanasia. These can be difficult to locate, and their worth is highly contentious, yet it brings to the fore the demand for information on ending one's life in a manner that is quick and painless. Pressure is applied to Internet providers to close down these sites as if restricting information about suicide will reduce either the desire or action.

References

English, C., Olle, J., & Dwyer, J. (2015). Coroners Prevention Unit, Coroners Court of Victoria. See: Transcript of hearing to *Inquiry into End of Life Choices*, Melbourne, November 18, www.parliament.vic.gov.au/lsic/inquiries/article/2611.

Huxtable, R. (2013). *Euthanasia*. London: Hodder & Stoughton.

Kass, L. (1989). Neither for love nor money: Why doctors must not kill. *Public Interest, 94*(Winter). See https://www.nationalaffairs.com/storage/app/uploads/public/58e/1a4/df3/58e1a4df371cf970949562.pdf.

Tatz, A. (2010). *Dangerous disease and dangerous therapy: Principles and practice*. Southfield, MI: Targum Press Inc.

Verhofstadt, M., Thiennport, L., & Peters, G.-J. Y. (2017). When unbearable suffering incites psychiatric patients to request euthanasia: Qualitative study. *British Journal of Psychiatry, 211*(4), 238–245.

---

[7]https://exitinternational.net/about-exit/history/.

Chapter 11
The Coroners

Coroner: an official whose duty is to enquire, on behalf of the king, how any violent death was occasioned, for which purpose a jury of twelve persons is impanelled.

—Samuel Johnson's *Dictionary*, 1755

There are a few who envy me. They want to know what they have to do to get my job, to be who I am. 'It's only death, how hard can it be?' Here, I silently reply, take it all. Every festering remnant of the people no one cared about in life, much less in death; all the broken children who will never know that I had grieved for them. Take it all. Just leave me my car keys so I can go home permanently. Someone else can listen to the bullshit Death loves to spew. He never shuts up.

—Joseph Scott Morgan [A former medical examiner in Louisiana and Georgia, USA]

Abstract The office of coroners and medical examiners; standards of proof required for suicide verdicts; some bizarre rulings on suicide; who is appointed to coronial positions; the matter of under-reporting of suicide; Australian research findings on suicide determinations.

Keywords Coroners and medical examiners · Rulings on suicide

In Britain and in her former colonies, the coroner is a somewhat mysterious but impressive official who conducts another seemingly quaint ritual from yesteryear—an inquisition or inquest. In America, that official is called a medical examiner, usually shortened to ME. The glamourised nature of this office was celebrated in the Canadian television series *Wojeck* in the 1960s, *Quincy M.E.*, the American television series of 1976–1983 and in Patricia Cornwell's popular thrillers featuring Kay Scarpetta, an M.E. and something of a forensic anthropologist. In Britain, in 2015, a mediocre television series, *The Coroner*, didn't do much for the profession. The 1990s Australian television programme, *State Coroner*, was a much more credible

© Springer Nature Switzerland AG 2019
C. Tatz and S. Tatz, *The Sealed Box of Suicide*,
https://doi.org/10.1007/978-3-030-28159-5_11

and serious effort to portray this profession. As to forensic pathology, the British television series *Silent Witness* may have entertained millions with its gore and its Sherlock Holmesian dissectors, but the depiction was of a quite unreal and aberrant mortuary.

The forensic parts in Herbert Lieberman's 1976 novel, *City of the Dead*, is a highwater mark of works on the universe of medical examiners. He began his book with what he described as 'an old adage':

> The psychiatrist knows all and does nothing
>
> The surgeon knows nothing and does all.
>
> The dermatologist knows nothing and
>
> does nothing.
>
> The pathologist knows everything,
>
> But a day too late.

The first formal mention of the notion of 'coroner' was in the year 1194. In mediaeval England, justices travelled along the 'Eyre', the name given to the judicial circuit. Their job was to hold 'the pleas of the crown', that is, to hold court, inspect villages, settle disputes and impose fines. By 1194, this system had become inefficient and crooked: in the long time it took the justices to travel, local sheriffs waxed fat by squeezing the peasants and not collecting revenue for the king.

The bureaucrat Walter Hubert established a new unit of officials charged with 'keeping the pleas of the crown' (*custos placitorum coronae*). The new coroners (or 'Crowners' as they were long called) documented the claims the king could make. They promoted the king's rights and interests, including 'taking care' of discovered treasure or valuables washed ashore. They took an interest in the violent deaths in homicide and suicide because their estates were inevitably forfeitable to the crown (as discussed in Chap. 3).

Today, a coroner's responsibility is, among other things, to explain how and why sudden deaths have occurred, to allay suspicions and fears, to hold public agencies to account for the deaths of those who died in their custody, to improve public health and safety and to reinforce the rule of law (Dillon and Hadley 2015: 2). This official also investigates and certifies deaths relating to disasters. In America, an M.E. has similar but not quite the same role as a coroner: their M.E. investigates unusual or suspicious deaths or injuries and in many state jurisdictions performs post-mortem autopsies.

11.1 Who Are Appointed

Appointments vary from country to country and within countries. There is little consistency on qualifications for the position. Many states now insist on legally or medically qualified persons, often magistrates, but several jurisdictions appoint people who have no such qualifications. In some regions, the office is an elected one.

In the Australian state of Victoria, all magistrates are deemed qualified as coroners but not all of them do coronial work. They usually undergo a two-week coronial training course. Perhaps 10% of their workloads involve coronial matters. Some 90% of these cases do not go to inquest and, in non-inquest matters in the non-metropolitan regions, clerks of petty sessions write up the findings. As in New South Wales, there is a full-time State Coroner and two full-time senior coroners.

In the UK, some jurisdictions require the coroner to be medically or legally qualified or to have both qualifications. In some US jurisdictions, the office of coroner is considered a prize, earned through a hard-fought electoral contest. Few untrained people occupy these positions. For the larger cities, coroners are appointed as medical examiners, that is, they are salaried, qualified and accredited forensic pathologists. In smaller towns, justices of the peace act as coroners and inevitably refer 'uncertain' cases to a forensic pathologist, either locally or in the nearest larger city. In cities like Dallas, the medical examiner has several death investigators, men and women with university degrees as well as on-the-job training. They work to, and for, the medical examiner and have co-equal access to death and crime scenes with police.

The now discarded *Coroners Act* of New South Wales provided for a State Coroner in Sydney and 'assistant coroners' in rural centres. The assistants were, in fact, clerks of petty sessions, minor semi- or quasi-judicial officials charged with such matters as registering marriages, births and deaths, land titles, issuing licences and the like. They were also the local coroners and handled suicides in most cases, surrendering the 'difficult' ones to Sydney head office. Between 1997 and 1999, Colin Tatz interviewed some 34 such clerks: one had a degree and several had not finished high school. Some had undergone a two-day in-service training course, others had no training at all but 'learned on the job'. The majority acknowledged their Catholic or lapsed Catholic adherence and signified that they regarded suicide as a cardinal sin and would, where possible, render an open or accident verdict rather than subject a family to shame and stigma. This was under-reporting at its worst.

Magistrate Hugh Dillon, former deputy chief coroner in New South Wales, studied coronial practices in Germany, Canada and England in 2015 (Dillon 2015). Even the new coronial system in that state was inadequate:

> To be blunt, while coronial services in NSW perform well in some respects, there are significant defects and inefficiencies that are actually or potentially costly to grieving families and the public interest. (These comments apply to varying extents to other Australian jurisdictions as well.) A striking feature of the Ontario system is respect for the people of Ontario. This is evidenced both by the government investment in excellent facilities, and the ser-

vices' commitment to excellence. In contrast, a striking feature of the NSW coronial system is that government's recurrent expenditure per case on coronial services is half the national average and second lowest in the Commonwealth. NSW Health is making significant efforts to improve forensic pathology services but the Department of Justice is not matching its commitment. The professional commitment to excellence of individual coroners can be found in NSW but facilities and systems provided by government have fallen well short of best practice and way behind those provided by other major states, especially in Victoria and Queensland. Some important improvements could be achieved at little or no cost to government.

In New Zealand, before 1988, no formal legal or medical qualifications were required for coronial appointments. Coroners included an accountant, and a publican in a small town who was also the fire chief. In the main, private practice barristers and solicitors were appointed and were independent of government service. Each had an inquest officer, a police constable, who assisted in collecting evidence. The Law Commission Report of 2000 described the coronial system as 'the poor relation of the justice system'.[1] But Colin Tatz worked with several of these men and found the system, however flawed in the eyes of the Law Commmission, a great deal more professional than the New South Wales system then in operation.

Their system changed with new legislation in 2006. Under the new Coroners Act, all coroners are appointed as tenured judicial officers. They must have at least five years experience in practice. Today, the 18 full-time coroners have an average of 19 years post-qualification experience, certainly more time in office than occurs in Australia. Judges of the District Court are ex-officio coroners but usually don't act as such.

The Canadian coroner in Iqaluit, the capital of Nunavut (where Colin Tatz conducted fieldwork) was a trained lawyer and a government official. Admittedly, Nunavut has a small Inuit population (some 38,000 persons) but the coroner had his finger on every case, by name, detail and circumstance. He, perhaps uniquely, kept tabs on the Inuit statistics and did his best to inform other government agencies and visiting researchers of the patterns he was discerning. His function and his involvement made him an integral part of the suicide picture, which was vivid enough.

For a very long period in England, the coroner had to be a barrister or solicitor or a medical practitioner of some five years standing. The M.E. system was, and remains, quite mixed in terms of the qualifications required. In France, the official is the *Médecin légiste,* in Italy, the *Medicina legale*, in Germany, the *Gerichtmediziner*. In Spain and Portugal, investigative forensic pathologists work under the supervision of an examining magistrate. In Greece, a coroner is *iiatrodikastis*, a medical judge.

In Australia, there are eight jurisdictions (six states and two territories) each with its own coronial system and each with its own qualifications for that office. Today, the practice in each jurisdiction is to appoint magistrates as coroners, with

---

[1]Law Commission Report 62 Coroners (2000: xi).

magistrates defined as 'Australian lawyers'. But, as discussed in Chap. 12, Australian law curricula have no formal units of study in coronial law and jurisprudence. In practice, they too 'learn on the job'.

11.2 The Matter of Presumption

The main role of coroners is to determine the cause of death. By convention, suicide has to be proved. It may not be presumed, even in the most obvious cases. And therein lies an enormous problem, namely, that there is a great deal more suicide out there than is reflected in official statistics. Since most matters relating to suicide are based on official statistics, a modicum of accuracy is essential.

There are three categories of presumption in law: those that cannot be rebutted by contrary evidence, those that are rebuttable, and presumptions of fact that a judge or jury may draw from other proven facts. In most coronial systems, suicide *may not be presumed at all*. That dictum stems from case precedents, not from statutes prohibiting presumption. Freckelton and Ranson (2006: 634) noted that the Ontario High Court stressed that the presumption against suicide is 'rooted in the general conviction that a finding of suicide is grave in the highest degree and its consequences are serious'—hence, no presumption is permitted. The origins of *graveness* and *seriousness* stem from the days when suicide was deemed criminal and therefore required levels of proof beyond 'the balance of probabilities'. It also arose from family appeals against coronial verdicts that the appellants believed caused them shame or stigma, or loss of life-insurance payouts which often contained clauses excluding suicide or suicide within, say, a year of the policy's operation.

Coroners have a unique power: only they can determine a formal verdict of suicide. Police, ambulance staff, doctors, paramedics, hospital and prison personnel—those who may well be the first to sight a deceased in situ have no say in the determination. But this rather strange restriction on presumption, even in the face of clear-cut signs, leads to a skewing of the statistics on suicidal deaths. This dictum of non-presumption arose not from statutes but from the precedent of a British case of 1912: *R v HM Coroner for the City of London*. The Chief Justice ruled that a coronial presumption of suicide, however strongly suggested, by a man who had climbed over an 'effective railing' on the roof garden of his apartment and fallen, was invalid:

> If a person dies a violent death, the possibility of suicide may be there for all to see but it must not be presumed merely because it seems on the face of it to be a likely explanation. Suicide must be proved by evidence, and if it is not proved by evidence it is the duty of the coroner not to find suicide, but to find an open verdict.

What underlay this decision was the determination of a widow not only to preclude the very notion that her husband took an early exit but to exclude any possible stigma on her good family name. More of this is treated below.

11.3 Suicide Statistics

The American scholar Stefan Timmermans (2005) has studied the vexed question of whether suicide statistics are so biased as to be valueless or are of sufficient quality to be of worth. The matter of reporting and under-reporting was addressed by Durkheim more than a century ago. For us, the broad statistics are just that—broad indicators of a broad set of trends, broad enough to indicate a simple upwards or downwards movement or a steady state of affairs. But the statistics are crucial for the preventionists and for the interested general public. It is the preventionists who are wedded to targets and targets are contingent on the official rates of suicide.

Timmermans raised the important question of the 'hidden' suicides, those that may be designated as accidental or of unknown cause, particularly among such cohorts as adolescents, the elderly, some ethnic minorities, pedestrians, and single-vehicle road deaths.

We have talked at some length about stigma and shame and the good intentions of many coroners who want to avoid upsetting families unduly and so find an alternative semi-satisfactory verdict. (We discuss family reactions below). But Timmermans was insightful when he argued that the professionalism of coroners and M.E.s is attacked often enough to put pressure on them to be conservative in their determinations. The quotation from Joseph Morgan at the head of this chapter indicates a high level of frustration felt by those who investigate death.

Below, we discuss several examples of bizarre coronial rulings that have derived from the dictum of non-presumption. What is significant for the study of suicide is that there are a great many more self-deaths than those that are determined by proof that satisfies coroners and medical examiners.

11.4 Standards of Proof

The *James Maughan* case in Britain in 2018 ruled that a civil standard rather than a criminal standard of proof of suicide is now sufficient for coroners to determine suicide, that is, a change from a 98 to 99% standard down to a 51% level. Australian coroners operate on the civil standard—the balance of probabilities—but with the application of the *Briginshaw* principle enunciated by Justice Sir Owen Dixon in a 1938 divorce case. He ruled that many matters of judgment are not amenable to precise quantitative calibration. What is needed is a comfortable level of satisfaction or actual persuasion, having regard to the significance of what is under consideration and the inherent likelihood or otherwise of it having occurred. *Briginshaw* is thus a sliding scale to suicide findings in the contemporary Australian coronial system (Dillon and Handley 2015: 113; Jowett 2018). Generally, Briginshaw has come to mean something in the vicinity of a 75% standard of proof. Briginshaw is invoked if the 'the seriousness of an allegation' or 'the gravity of the consequences' seems necessary to reach 'a reasonable satisfaction' for a verdict. The 'gravity of the consequences' has been seen to lie in such effects as an impact on a family of a suicide verdict, again the shroud of shame underlying the determination processes.

11.5 Some Coronial Rulings

Suicide is not simply, or even complexly, that which appears in the statistics. It is also about that which doesn't appear, that is, the cases that are almost certainly suicide but were not declared as such by the coronial system. We will, of course, never know just how many fall into that category. A few such examples will suffice here.

In a New South Wales town in 1998, the local coroner wrote: 'Z died as a result of Alcohol and Amitriptyline intoxication, however, I am not satisfied on the evidence that the deceased intended to take her life'. The attending police officer had submitted the required procedural form in which he wrote: 'It would appear that the deceased wife of a policeman had become depressed on Friday night and on this Saturday night had drunk two bourbons and taken a quantity of tablets with the intent to take her life. A torn up note was located in the rubbish bin which indicates this intention' (Tatz 2005: 53).

In another town, population 1,130 and one doctor, two Aboriginal girls were given prescriptions for the analgesic paracetamol. Both swallowed whole packets, both died, and both cases were ruled as accidental death, with the postscript that both may have been illiterate and couldn't read the warning notices. Relatives were adamant that both girls had talked about finding exit strategies. They had also been 'doctor-shopping' in nearby towns. In the name of such misconceived kindness, the suicide pattern and picture become distorted.

Early in 2016, the New Zealand press suggested that the suicide rate in that country may well be three times greater than the official reports indicated. This followed the death of an artist in Wellington, seemingly by her own hand and with a note on a pad beside her bed. There wasn't evidence enough, ruled the coroner, to prove whether she was then 'mentally capable of forming an intention to take her life' (*Sunday Star Times*, 29 May 2016). Intent, the *mens rea* is a quintessential element of a crime; crucial to both indictment and verdict. But suicide is no longer a crime—so why must there be such adamant insistence on mental health capacity, why the need for 'clear and unequivocal', 'clear and cogent' evidence in self-death cases? It no longer makes sense.

In the USA, we have some equally bizarre rulings highlighted by Timmermans (2005: at 319–326). Guy Dubos, a White male, was found dead in his apartment. He had problems with a recent divorce, was filing for bankruptcy, was a recovering alcoholic, had a diabetic insulin pump attached to his stomach; there were bottles of antidepressants to hand, and he had left three poetic-style notes indicating a suicidal intention. The lengths to which relatives went to obviate a suicide verdict were astonishing. The insulin pump accidentally 'overdosed' him but because insulin breaks down in short time, one couldn't say for certain that it was deliberate or accidental. The notes were presented as 'amateur dabbling in poetry', and 'poets tend to be a morbid kind'. With challenges left, right and centre, and with new forensic pathologists appointed, the outcome—despite a pathology finding of low level heart disease—was 'cardiac arrythmia' and therefore declared a 'natural' death.

Andy Williams was a White male in his 30s, diagnosed as bipolar, with a history of threatening to jump, and on at least one occasion had to be talked down from jumping off a water tower in a mental health facility (on the promise of a McDonald's 'happy meal'). He talked of his suicidal thoughts and his desire to harm himself. On an ill-advised family outing, Andy 'fell' over a fifth-floor parking garage railing, deemed high enough to avert any toppling possibilities. The family fought all the way to have his death deemed accidental. The father declared that he simply couldn't live with a suicide determination. The rest of the family said that the moral stigma of suicide was too great and was 'a personal affront' and there could be no public health benefit that outweighed their personal suffering.

Timmermans raised the matter of suicide deniers. The literature on fluoride deniers, smoking deniers, vaccination deniers and climate change deniers is replete with conspiracy theories, 'fake news', the diabolic and the devilish. But with the suicide variety, there are only the highly personal factors of love of the deceased and the senses of stigma, not real stigma, for the living: the Williams son is dead and the father can't live with his manner of death.

How often such way out rulings occur is something we don't know. Sifting through all the files at the NSW State Coroners Court, many cases recorded single-vehicle deaths on good roads and in calm weather conditions, on occasion with rosary beads in one hand, hitting the only tree on the wrong side of the road and without skid marks. The majority were ruled as 'accidental' deaths. Short of a 'suicide cold case' unit of the police, we will never know.

Of interest is the contextual opposite. Phoebe Handsjuck died by falling down a garbage chute in a high-rise apartment building. The family wanted the verdict changed, and in 2018, the state of Victoria in Australia enacted a statute allowing, for the first time ever, challenges to coronial findings, a result, in part, of Phoebe's case. Her death was deemed suicide but police now believe it may have been murder.

A recent Canadian study of regional variations in suicide (Renaud et al 2018) found significant variations as between provinces and territories, with decreased rates in some and increased rates in others. They attributed the differences to divergent legislation on prevention strategies and urged more consistency. This study, like so many others, assumed that all coronial reporting systems are of a gold standard and are consistent—which, of course, they are not, as discussed below.

11.6 The Matter of Grief

There is another facet to stigma avoidance, another example of benevolent intent for the sake of a deceased's family and friends: the 'therapeutic coroner', those 'who care too much' (Carpenter et al. 2015; Tait and Carpenter 2013). In an earlier chapter, we described the responses of the New York M.E. to the kin of those who 'fell' rather than 'jumped' from the inferno of the Twin Towers in 2001. *The Times* of London (6 January 2017) reported that the under-reporting in the UK may be as high as 50%—mostly 'to give comfort to grief-stricken families'. The stigma of the Middle Ages hovers over all suicides in the West and affects the work of coroners.

But the 'caringness' of coroners, those who find the comforting euphemisms of 'misadventure', 'accidental death' and 'open verdict' has another basis, namely, grief. Unlike the *DSM*, which is almost dismissive of the notion of prolonged grief, here we have legal officers recognising that, in the absence of readily accessible grief counselling, the bereaved in suicide cases need a great deal of solace, consolation that takes the form of finding a kinder way of explaining a deceased's end of life. Australian psychiatrist Beverley Raphael in her *Anatomy of Bereavement* (1983) stated that suicide bereavement often leads to aggression and anger. Someone has to deal with that. And so, we arrive at the Hugh Dillon and Margaret Hadley text—*The Australasian Coroners' Manual* (2015). Their third chapter is entitled 'The bereaved and their grief', with 27 pages devoted to how coroners should handle the experience of grief and grief across cultures and ethnicities. That we find remarkable for its sensibility and sensitivity. But there can be no doubting that coronial/M.E. care about people leads to a masking of the real suicide numbers.

11.7 Australian Research on Suicide Determinations

The Australian Research Council allocates funding on a competitive basis to academic research at universities. In 2015, Belinda Carpenter, Gordon Tait, Diego de Leo and Colin Tatz were awarded a major grant to investigate coronial determinations of suicide as a category of death. The findings, due for reporting in 2019, are summarised here in the words of the chief investigator, law Professor Belinda Carpenter of the Queensland University of Technology:

> Interviews with 32 coroners in Australian states and territories [except Tasmania[2]] revealed that there were three inter-related areas that caused coroners the most concern with respect to suicide and the law: definitions of suicide; clarity of intent; and the legal standard of proof. In these areas, consistency in approach within and across jurisdictions could be improved through law reform as well as training that takes into account the current state of knowledge as derived from the literature on suicide and self-harm.
>
> First, it was found that coroners differ significantly in terms of the definition of suicide they apply in practice, if one is employed at all. This has the likely implication that deaths may be treated very differently depending upon the coroner who makes the finding. This leads to the recommendation that, as there is currently no clear legal definition of suicide in any of the Coroners Acts, this needs to be rectified.
>
> Second, and despite variance in suicide definitions, discerning intent was agreed by most coroners to be the central issue in suicide determinations. Coroners appear well versed in the evidence that needs to be gathered when considering suicide as a legal finding, with many of the issues raised by coroners in interviews supported in the literature on suicide risk factors. However, it was found that coroners relied overly on certain risk factors and methods to indicate intent; and were inconsistent around key determinants of capacity, especially concerning age, alcohol and mental illness. It was identified that clarification of the law and/or training around particular elements that could be considered to fall within a suicide definition may contribute to greater consistency in approach.
>
> Third, it was revealed that coroners vary considerably on their application of the standard of proof required to reach a finding of suicide. This further supports a recommendation made in an earlier paper by the authors that the law guiding the application of standard of proof in suicide findings needs to be clarified in order to move towards nationally consistent approaches.
>
> There are a number of further conclusions to be drawn from this research with regard to the role of the Coroner. First, suicide rates are not simply an objective reflection of social truth. They are the product of a complex set of variables that inform and shape the coronial decision-making process. Probably the most significant of these is an ongoing unresolved tension within the role of coroner, a tension between their duty to produce defensible death statistics, and the effects of what has been referred to as 'therapeutic jurisprudence'—the belief that coroners should take some responsibility for the emotional wellbeing of the bereaved families. The most visible effect of this unresolved element of coronial practice is a significant downward pressure on suicide rates.
>
> Second, Indigenous [Aboriginal] Australian families are treated differently within the coronial system. There appears to be far less reticence in reaching a finding of suicide if the deceased is Indigenous. Therefore, while Indigenous suicide rates are clearly unacceptably high, it may well be that part of the disparity between those figures and non-Indigenous Australia is a greater coronial reluctance to reach a finding of suicide for the non-Indigenous. There is also a circularity in reasoning by coroners, who anticipate a higher suicide rate among Indigenous Australians, and are then part of the mechanism of its production.

These are not 'happy' findings but poor tidings for a coronial system that is believed to have transformed in the past decade. The coronial training aspect of these findings will be treated in the next chapter on professions.

---

[2]The only jurisdiction that declined participation in the study.

What needs comment here is the finding on Aboriginal suicide. The Australian health system is characterised by entrenched racism. Our experience and the national data sets indicate that 'closing-the-gap' between Aboriginal and non-Aboriginal health outcomes is stifled by racism and what we see is a case of conscious or unconscious racial profiling. An anticipatory stereotyping that first, Aborigines fore-mostly *do* rather than *may* commit suicide; second, Aboriginal people are less likely to react badly to such a finding and hence are more accepting of verdicts, less likely to create waves in the name of protecting family honour.

11.8 Relevant Matters: Detection

Importantly, there is thus far no unanimity about some issues: first, the need for coroners to have a dedicated and regular (and not random) police unit attached to them as investigators; second, the need for a formal course or qualification in coronial studies, not only for coroners but for police, all judicial officers, prison personnel and hospital staff, a matter we have been advocating for more than a decade.

Detection is a problem. The lack thereof can only lie in three processes: the initial reporting by a police patrol called to a home or an institution because the death is not overtly natural or is in some way suspicious; the hospital and medical staff where a patient has died for no seemingly (progressive or reasonable) reason following treatment or surgery; a coronial 'blockage' or unwillingness to determine suicide.

In most unnatural or suspicious deaths, it is the police who are the first port of call. They report the scene and the surrounds; they observe and record evidence; they take depositions from witnesses or kin; they report their assembled files to the coroner. The coroner is the adjudicator, so to speak: he or she is not the death investigator in situ, nor the initial 'detective' on the scene. Given the apparent concern expressed by both governments and the community for suicide prevention, it would not be outlandish for governments to fund dedicated suicide units in their police forces rather than randomly assign personnel doing the rounds of police work. The New Zealand Police have implemented that.

In an earlier chapter, we quoted Joseph Zubin as saying that unravelling the cause of a suicide death post-mortem is well-nigh impossible. True, but a trained forensic anthropologist in a 'detection team' can do what nobody else can do or seems to want to do—understand the contextual life of the deceased.

References

Carpenter, B., Tait, G., Stobbs, N., & Barnes, M. (2015). When coroners care too much: Therapeutic jurisprudence and suicide findings. *Journal of Judicial Administration, 24*(3), 172–183.

Dillon, H. (2015). *Raising coronial standards of performance: Lessons from Canada, Germany and England*. Winston Churchill Memorial Trust of Australia. http://www.churchilltrust.com.au.

Dillon, H., & Handley, M. (2015). *The Australasian coroner's manual*. Sydney: The Freedom Press.

Freckelton, I., & Ranson, D. (2006). *Death investigation and the coroner's inquest*. Oxford: Oxford University Press.

Jowett, S., Carpenter, B., & Tait, G. (2018). Determining suicide under Australian law. *UNSW Law Journal, 41*(2).

Law Commission (New Zealand). (2000). Coroners, No. 62, Wellington: New Zealand.

Lieberman, H. (1976). *City of the dead*. Australia: Hutchinson.

Maughan Case. (2018). *R (Maughan) v HM Senior Coroner Oxfordshire and others* 26 July 2018.

Morgan, J. S. (2012). *Blood beneath my feet: The journey of a Southern death investigator*. Port Townsend, WA: Feral House.

R v HM Coroner for the City of London (1975), All England Law Reports [1975] 3 All ER: 538–540.

Raphael, B. (1983). *The anatomy of bereavement*. New York, NY: Basic Books Inc., Publishers.

Renaud, J., Lesage, A., Gagné, M., MacNeil, S., Légaré, G., Geoffroy, M.-C., Skinner, R., & McFaull, S. (2018). Regional Variations in Suicide and Undetermined Death Rates among Adolescents across Canada. *The Journal of the Canadian Academy of Child and Adolescent Psychiatry, 27*(2).

Tatz, C. (2005). *Aboriginal suicide is different: A portrait of life and self-destruction*. Canberra: Aboriginal Studies Press.

Timmermans, S. (2005). Suicide determination and the professional authority of medical examiners. *American Sociological Review, 70*(2), 311–333.

Chapter 12
The Professionals

We trust our health to the physician; our fortune and sometimes our life and reputation to the lawyer and attorney. Such confidence could not safely be reposed in people of a very mean and low condition. Their reward must be such, therefore, as may give them that rank in society which so important a trust requires. The long time and great expense which must be laid out in their education, when combined with this circumstance, necessarily enhances still further the price of their labour.

—Adam Smith [Scottish author of *Wealth of Nations* (1776), Book I, Chapter 10]

Most doctors are prisoners of their education and shackled by their profession.

—Richard Diaz [American radiation oncologist and author]

Abstract The trained professionals and the untrained amateurs who deal with suicide; the 'ownership' of a suicide problem and the role of ethnic community elders; the nature of cultural accommodation and a short discussion on physician's suicide.

Keywords Assumptions about knowledge · Cultural accommodation · Doctor suicide

In many Western societies, the tenor of the tabloids is that suicide is at crisis point, that governments aren't doing enough, that more money is needed for mental health… Here the cry is that the Australian Aboriginal communities have an even more disastrous 'epidemic' of self-destruction. If one assumes [and we don't] the aberrant and contagious nature of suicide, apart from funding matters, the more profound question is who will do the preventing or the intervening, who will provide deliverance? An obvious answer in many, but not all cases, is the professionals.

The hallmark of the professional is that they are qualified, certificated and authorised to practise a profession or a trade, a permit that demonstrates that the person is learned, competent, experienced and skilled. The validating authority formally pronounces the person as proficient in a particular field, and the signed and sealed certificate on the wall is testament to the service-seeker that all is well and that trust, above all, is warranted. But certification is not always a guarantee of professionalism, of knowledge, skills or competence.

The self-dead are the province of coroners, the living that of the medicine persons. We have seen how little training and tuition there is for the profession of coroner. So what instruction does the medical profession—in general and in particular—have about suicide? What of the adjunct service providers such as the nurses, social workers, occupational therapists, the policy-makers and the bureaucrats? We also address the phenomenon of physician suicide—not only because their suicide rate is high but because their exits are always accompanied by explanatory causal factors that have little to do with 'mental illness', an interpretation and a mitigation that is rarely accorded to other suiciders.

Oncologist Richard Diaz contends that most doctors are prisoners of their education and are shackled by their profession. *Constrained* may be an apt term for those wedded and welded to the 'mental illness' model of suicide, but to say that they are imprisoned by their education is to infer that they had an education about suicide. A wrong inference, as often enough the professionals are amateurs in the matter of suicide.

We describe the Australian mental health system as having four tiers of professionals. Tier I includes psychiatrists and medical practitioners—in both the private and public systems—who are licensed to practise what they do. Tier II has licensed and registered clinical psychologists and mental health nurses in both the public and private sectors. Tier III embraces the social workers, speech pathologists, peer workers, mentors, counsellors and technical college-trained and certificated personnel. Quite separately in Tier IV, we have non-government organisation (NGO) workers, advisers and policy people, mostly educated but often professionally unqualified persons who work in the areas of stigma, awareness, mental health policy, media guidelines and public campaigns, again in both the private and public sectors.

There are many in these tiers who have formal qualifications but who were untrained, and remain so, in matters of suicide and even in mental health. 'Learning on the job' is a repeated rationalisation, but suicide is hardly a matter of an apprenticeship in laying bricks or building bookshelves.

One aspect of the professionals is that they often tend to have a monopoly on knowledge and a monopoly on the supply of services. In Herbert Lieberman's *City of the Dead* (1976: 17), which we quoted earlier, his coronial investigator makes the telling point that 'doctors, just like clergymen, have an obligation to at least pretend to a wisdom they don't really possess'. Thus, in Tier I, only GPs and psychiatrists can prescribe medications, and only limited specialisations can order diagnostic testing and scanning procedures under Medicare, the national public health insurance scheme. In Australia, at least, the referral system—by which only the general practitioners at the bottom of the hierarchy are allowed to refer patients upwards into a hierarchy of knowledge specialists—indicates the deference pyramid. Medical and other specialisations are recognised (and endorsed) by the state, which in turn empowers them in a variety of ways, including the ways that give them rank in society. They often exclude female competition, or downgrade it, and they stand apart from those who have good social knowledge of situations. In this sense, professionals are in occupations that are based on advanced or complex or esoteric or arcane knowledge (Macdonald 1995: 1).

Medical specialists have a different power to that of legal specialists. The latter often help fashion systems and protocols and work within governmental and parliamentary systems. But it is only the medicine specialist who can fix the leaking aorta, save the stroke victim from paralysis, ease the lung cancer, control the diabetes, remove the cataracts and keep the human machine at work and in a sociable condition. They are 'the straighteners who unbend the crooked', who heal the sick, who keep the well even weller. In that sense, they are beyond monopoly.

We like to think of the professions as goodly and godly, virtuous people who do what they do for the benefit of mankind, humanity, ever repairing a flawed world. We tend to invest them with more morality and less concern about 'enhancing the price of their labour'. Doctors and nurses regularly top 'most trusted profession' surveys. Society often recognises a small group of kindred spirits as the 'helping professions'.

12.1 Degrees of Learning

Given the high-rank order of deaths by suicide, one would think that suicide education, of whatever kind, would be reasonably high in the curricula of doctors and nurses. Not so.

Some 15 years ago, a young psychiatry registrar at a Sydney university asked Colin Tatz to participate in a weekend live-in seminar on suicide—because, she said, she and her colleagues had had no training about the complex psychosocial, traumatic consequences and cultural aspects of suicide and were about to embark on practice. Some 40 registrars attended lectures and tutorials from three psychiatry professors—Louise Newman, Ernest Hunter, the late Beverley Raphael, and Colin Tatz. There was no shortage of material for that 12-hour face-to-face tuition. One would have thought that suicide education had improved since then. Not so.

In most of Australia's 43 universities, a unit of study is of one-semester duration (13 weeks) entailing 39 hours of face-to-face teaching, that is, two one-hour lectures and a one-hour tutorial or practical demonstration class (at least) each week. Recent online forms of teaching may be calculated in other ways. Until the 1980s, most course units were of two-semester length. Nevertheless, a great deal can be achieved by both teacher and pupil in the one-semester time frame.

We engaged with a great many medical practitioners. Their answers to a casual question about how much they were taught about suicide, or about mental health, were a shock. Answers ranged from zero to recollection of a 50-minute lecture somewhere along the way. Too casual, we thought, and so we approached teaching staff at Sydney's two largest tertiary institutions, Sydney University and the University of New South Wales (UNSW), both in the top 50 of world university rankings. Their responses, presented anonymously here, tell a particular tale:

> Short answer is very little. Students will get a lecture on suicide as part of their psychiatry rotation. When they do their clinical attachments, suicidal and self-harming behaviour are talked about as part of a risk assessment and they may come into contact with NSW Health documents – clinical pro-formas called 'MH-OAT' – that provide check-lists to complete as against a nuanced risk evaluation of the patient. Certainly no Durkheim or Baechler in that situation. If anything it is Bob [Robert] Goldney's orthodoxy of 'depression, depression, depression' – his so-called 'Real Estate Analogy'.

Sydney once had a reading in a mental health ethics course on the Japanese perspective on suicide as part of a week on 'autonomy', but this was replaced for a topic-based consideration of 'physician assisted suicide'. Another professor 'touches on youth suicide' in his week in that unit, but not much else.

A UNSW staffer taught suicide, a lecture which focused particularly on clinical assessment, to phase 3 medical students doing psychiatry. The lecture was of 45 minute duration. That academic also taught suicide to phase 2 medical students doing women's and child health under the rubric of mental health ('mental disorders and suicide prevention among young Australians'). That session took 90 minutes. The former was core content. The second was not (the subject of suicide was introduced as an example/avenue for talking about the topic of mental health).

Nurse training is a similar story. One major Queensland university teacher had this to say:

> I teach a grad dip/masters in mental health. We do cover suicide in that course, but the numbers are small, as postgraduate study for nurses is expensive and not mandatory in mental health services. This study is also online (much to my chagrin).
>
> At undergraduate level we have one short lecture on suicide. I can't speak for the whole of Australia — There are about 36 schools of nursing, and each have their own curriculum.
>
> University of Wollongong and Southern Cross University have a good complement of mental health lecturers and they may cover this in more depth there.
>
> I suspect that such a topic is better taught when nurses and doctors are actually practising (rather than learning at uni) (via professional development) because they may realise how pertinent it is to practise then.

To this, we can add the information that the curriculum for psychiatric nurse training no longer teaches its earlier core course on mental health.

There is no need of a survey of all medical and nursing schools to find out how much or how little they teach in these fields. There is enough evidence to say that it is abysmal—given the prominence of suicide on the public agenda and given the sovereignty of the healing professions on the matter of suicide. The vehemence with which some in the medical and allied professions assert that suicide is solely, or mainly, an outcome of mental ill-health suggests that practitioners of all kinds have had solid and focused tuition and training, that they are well versed in the history of suicide, its aetiology, manifestation, its role, place and legacy in a society, in its mitigation, alleviation, even prevention. If there is any validity to the view that one in four (or five) persons in a Western population like that of America and Australia are suffering from some type of 'mental disorder', one would expect that training in the healing professions would be intense. Most medical specialisations take up to seven years, with at least two or three years of post-bachelor degree study that involves internship, a registrarship and examinations. Given the universality of that kind of curriculum, one has to note that 'mental illness' is usually very much less than a semester's duration and that a specific suicide focus ranges from zero exposure to a fifty-minute lecture. [Coronial law and practice feature not at all.]

The rationalisation that doctors in general practice 'learn on the job' about suicide makes no sense at all. What is to be learned? On presentation of suicide ideation, or talk of early demise, the GP usually does one of two things: prescribes antidepressants or refers the patient to a psychiatrist or psychologist. There is little, if any, learning involved. [Worth noting is that data from the Pharmaceutical Benefits Scheme shows that in 2017 one in eight Australians was on antidepressants, including 100,000 children under 17.]

The message, at least in Australia, is that if you experience suicidal thoughts (or mental health concerns) then immediately see a GP. In what other professions can we find so meagre a basis for so central a say and a sway in society?

In the case of Australian lawyers, a few of whom go on to be magistrates and then coroners, there are no units of study on coronial law and jurisprudence. One large Sydney university, offering a prestigious law degree, has an elective unit of study called 'Health Law' in which the role and place of coroner get some short place. The Dunedin coroner in New Zealand has sought the introduction of three coronial topics in a similar elective at Otago University.[1]

12.2 The Aboriginal Case

The Australian Aboriginal case is of interest here, for a number of reasons. Not the least of them is the conundrum of who 'owns' suicide? When suicide is a major

---

[1] Personal communication with Law Dean and Coroner.

factor in any one society or community does this mean that group 'owns' or has to 'own' that problem? To the exclusion of everyone else?

Yes, there is a propensity for Aboriginal communities to say that suicide is their problem and they have to contain it, as we saw earlier from an Inuit elder. But suicide has been a factor in Inuit society for a very long time, and the Australian Aboriginal experience of it is a very short one, some 60 years now.

Aboriginal 'autonomy', of a kind, dates from the early 1970s, hardly time to recover rights, rites, rituals, internal medical and pharmaceutical systems, infant survival and myriad other consequences of their genocide and then their incarceration on government settlements and church mission stations. The older patterns of malaria, leprosy, tuberculosis, dysentery, trachoma and gastro-enteritis have been replaced by a new reign of strokes, cardiac, renal, metabolic and cancer diseases. Isolation, social and physical, remains, as does endemic racism, poverty, unemployment, almost total reliance on social welfare benefits, neglect, second-class services and, too often, no services at all. There are very few public psychiatrists at all and even fewer living and working in Aboriginal communities in Australia.

In such circumstances, how does a community come to 'own' an almost alien set of behaviours that have arisen essentially from factors not of their making? We have said that suicide arises from the social order: yes, it also arises from social disorder, and many Aboriginal communities are in a state of dysfunction and disorder. Anthropologist Colin Turnbull, author of a major work on the Ik, the mountain people of East Africa, once explained that former hunter-gatherers, rounded up, relocated, made sedentary and changed from ordered societies to disordered ones; environments where the normal values of child-rearing, parental love and care, care of the young and aged, eroded. Kindness, care, love and reciprocity were, he said, the luxuries of ordered societies (Turnbull 1972).

Intentional or unconscious, there is an implication in mainstream attitudes to differentials in a longish list of social indicators. 'Closing-the-gap' was launched in 2007, a national programme aimed at reducing mortality, educational, health and social gaps, sometimes gulfs, between Aborigines and mainstream society. A dismal failure, for the most part, it aimed at 'better statistics' instead of addressing real people. An underlying feature of the programme was that eliminating or reducing deficits made *us* look better.

Twenty-year gaps in life expectancy didn't look good in a first-world democracy. Nor do eight- and 10-year old Aboriginal suicides.

Passing the suicide ball to Aboriginal persons is not appropriate and not an answer. There is something beyond the bizarre when we find that the professionals who claim sovereignty in this field then turn to a largely illiterate (in English) community to solve the problem. [In 1969 there were nine Aboriginal people at university; by 2017, the number of Aboriginal graduates was some 20,000, less than 3% of their population.] The rhetoric from government and clinicians is for Aboriginal 'empowerment' to address *their* suicide, a perverse demand from professionals who routinely *disempower* their patients. That there needs to be a partnership is certain. But more than partnership, there has to be an amalgam, not only of practical projects but in attitudes, as discussed below.

12.3 The Professional Amateurs

This oxymoron is used to identify a number of Aboriginal, Māori, Indian and Inuit elders who may lack formal Western education yet are the key decision-makers in their communities. Much of patriarchal dominance has gone, and it is matriarchal knowledge and direction that is in the forefront of holding groups intact. They are not merely 'talented amateurs' but skilled at marshalling the resistance and the resilience needed to survive both the societal and the geographic forces that, on the face of things, could have brought about their demise a long time ago.

What they have faced, and still face daily, is assimilation in the strict colonial sense of that word. It doesn't mean absorption of the smaller indigenous population into the larger White mainstream. Rather, it involves the ways in which colonial systems develop ideas, systems and institutions in their metropolitan centres and export them to the colonial outposts—in the belief that the locals *must* accommodate to these ideas. So, Madrid, Lisbon, London, Berlin, The Hague, Brussels and Rome evolved and developed educational, medical, engineering and architectural systems, exported them round the world and waited patiently, sometimes genocidally impatiently, for the locals to yield their systems in favour of the exports. We did this in Australia, and still do it: capital city ways of thinking and doing are sent out bush on the assumption that all is superior and the locals will take on the metropolitan wisdom, or else.

The 'good' colonial meaning of assimilation was not the extent to which the local communities accommodated to us, but the ways in which we, the exporters, accommodated to native ways of seeing and doing. The Portuguese did it best while imposing their language on African and Asian peoples. (They even encouraged inter-racial marriage.) Australian colonialism was based on the myth that there were no people before the British arrival in 1788, and that whatever human-like presence was there was but part and parcel of the native flora and fauna. Later, when that presence was on the verge of extirpation, came protection and with protection came the 'Jesus men', small coteries of public servants, poorly trained teachers, flying doctor services for rescue, fly-in-fly-out medical services that never allowed the normal doctor–patient relationships to develop.

There are two kinds of history, at the very least. The first is internal and personal, the ingredients that form the very essence of an ethnicity like Aboriginality, Māoridom and Inuit being. These include the nature of, and attitudes to, life and death, the pleasures and agonies, the inheritance of traditional ways of rites and rituals, the imbibed folkways and idioms. These elements constitute their 'inside' story, one totally ignored, misread or misunderstood by the mainstream. The second is the record and aggregate of past events, the narratives in time, the chronicles of what has befallen them as a result of good and bad faith over centuries. The outside story is also a chronicle of three key factors that have loomed so large in Aboriginal history, namely, geographic isolation, legal exclusion and administrative neglect.

To date, certainly until a decade ago, it was Aboriginal communities that had to be accommodating to the White way of doing things. 'Consultation', a widely touted practice, in effect meant not asking the people but telling the people what was to happen, especially in the health domain. Tuberculosis, gastro-enteritis and renal disease are one thing, suicide quite another. Recognising that, community elders have proclaimed, as we have seen earlier, that suicide is 'their problem', and they will take on the 'solutions'. But such ownership, such sovereignty is nowhere nearer to an answer to the enigma of suicide than is the Western, Anglo cohort of professionals. To insist that it is an 'indigenous problem' is also to walk away from it.

12.4   Suicide in the Medical Profession

The mantra of suicide prevention is '*if you have suicidal thoughts go see a doctor*'. Perversely, and tragically, the medical profession records above-average suicide rates in some countries. Why?

The data on medical suicides is inconsistent: the estimate of the number of doctors' suicides in America is between 300 and 400 annually. Writing in *The American Association for Physician Leadership*, health journalist Susan Kreimer (2018) reported that 'the suicide rate among doctors is somewhere between 28 and 40 per 100,000—or more than twice that of the overall population'. Anaesthetists and psychiatrists are at the higher risk (on the face of it because they have the readiest access to the means, Kreimer 2018). Presented at the American Psychiatric Association (APA) annual meeting in 2018, these figures showed that while female medical practitioners attempt suicide far less often than women in the general (American) population, their completion rate exceeded that of the general population by 2.5–4 times (the same as the completion rate of male doctors).

Pamela Wible is founder of what she calls 'the ideal medical care movement'. She is devoted to preventing physician suicides. Wible started keeping count of doctor suicides in 2012; by March 2018, she had registered 1,103 suicides. In her informative article, 'What I've learned from 1,103 doctor suicides', Wible detailed her conclusions (Wible 2017). She began with an historical perspective—high rates of suicide among doctors have been known for over 150 years, dating back to 1858. Yet despite this awareness, a century and a half later, 'the root causes of these suicides remain unaddressed'.

Today, the rates of physician suicide are so high that Wible proclaimed it a national health crisis with (her figures) a staggering one million Americans losing their doctor each year to suicide. For every female doctor who suicides, seven male doctors do so. Australian data show the female doctors suicide rate at 2.27 times the rate of the general population, male doctors slightly less often at 1.41 times the general population. Surveys of Australian medical students reported one in five experiencing suicidal ideation in the preceding 12 months (Swannell 2019a, b). The Australian Medical Association, in a submission on mandatory reporting laws (a mandatory responsibility to report a doctor if they are placing the public at risk of substantial harm because of impairment, such as mental health issue), outlined the situation:

> Doctors and other health workers have the highest suicide rate in Australia's White-collar workforce, according to data from the Australian National Coronial Information System. This shows that between January 1, 2011, and December 31, 2014, there were 153 health professionals who died as a result of suicide. Within the profession, that represented a suicide rate of 0.03 per cent, lower than for some occupations but the highest among White-collar workers. By raw numbers, more health professionals died by suicide in the three-year period than any other professional group.[2]

The Office for National Statistics, which covers England, recorded 430 health professionals who took their own lives between 2011 and 2015. Media reports from England in 2018 referred to a rise in doctor suicides with female doctors up to four times likely to suicide when compared to the general population.

The most common methods used by American doctors were poisoning and hanging. Wible found that female physicians prefered overdose while male physicians used firearms. Anaesthetists were at the highest risk, with overdose the most common method.

Location is significant. Physicians, it seems, chose to die where they've experienced their own pain. Doctors more often than not are found dead in their hospital call rooms; they jumped from hospital windows or shot themselves in hospital parking lots. They were found hanging in hospital chapels. Self-poisoning was the most common method according to a research paper by Hawton et al. (2000). For doctors, and retired doctors, barbiturates were the most commonly used means. 'Half of the anaesthetists who died used anaesthetic agents', a finding confirming that doctors have easy access to drugs and knowledge of which 'drugs and doses are likely to cause death'. The difference between suicide by doctors and the general population was method. Doctors self-poisoned and died of overdoses in greater proportions. The authors note that using medical drugs was also the commonest method for retired doctors. Of interest is this finding: while anaesthetists used anaesthetic agents, psychiatrists did not use psychotropic agents because they knew that psychotropic drugs were less likely to be fatal.

---

[2]The Australian Medical Association Submission (2017) on Mandatory Reporting can be found on their website: www.ama.com.au.

Are doctors more mentally unwell than the general population? Is there a neurological imbalance or serotonin deficiency more prevalent in psychiatrists and anaesthetists than in ophthalmologists or thoracic surgeons? Could doctors hide the warning signs better, able to suppress their suicidal intentions from their colleagues in ways non-medical people cannot?

Physician suicide is addressed extensively within medical associations. They list factors explaining why doctors suicide: stress; burn-out; long hours; bullying and harassment; limited time to deal with their own health issues; marriage and family break down; dealing with illnesses and death eating away at them; substance abuse; self-medication (and addiction); the constant threats (and reality) of litigation; complaints and malpractice; shame (being caught misusing drugs, sexual impropriety, criminal charges; careers stalling) and cultures that promoted income/profits over sensitive, time-consuming patient care.

Unlike the general population (with the possible exception of the military and politicians), doctors feared disclosing their own mental ill-health. Disclosure could result in suspension, restricted work practices, deregistration, shame and loss of livelihood. A secretive culture inhabits the medical sector. Revealing suicidal thoughts was a barrier discouraging doctors from seeking help. Dr. Ann McCormack, a staff specialist in endocrinology at Sydney's St Vincent's Hospital, offered a further explanation:

> What seems clear to me is that inherent traits in the individuals who choose a career in medicine, and often create excellent doctors, also set them up for high rates of distress. Perfectionism is rife among doctors. However, the very character trait that can contribute to success can also be a downfall in others. Maladaptive perfectionism refers to individuals experiencing distress over perceived personal or family failings (often unrealistic), and is associated with anxiety, depression, perceived burdensomeness and suicidal behaviour.

McCormack's contention, replicated in other discussions about physician suicide, suggests a personality trait in medical practitioners that is linked to high rates of burn-out and suicide. 'This Is Going To Hurt' (2017), Adam Kay's painfully humorous diary of being a junior doctor in the National Health System (England), makes this telling revelation following an attempted suicide by a medical colleague:

> There's a shared sense of numbness amongst the doctors. The only surprise is it doesn't happen more often – you're given huge responsibility, minimal supervision and absolutely no pastoral support. You work yourself to exhaustion, pushing yourself beyond what could be reasonably expected of you … In any other profession, if someone's job drove them to attempt suicide, you'd expect some kind of inquiry into what happened and a concerted effort to make sure it never happened again. Yet nobody said anything …. (Kay 2017: 106–107)

We are not aware of research delineating suicide rates between public and private doctors though we suspect the public health system takes a greater toll. Kay's book, part comedy part nightmare, portrayed a system that was ruthless on staff, driven by caring physicians operating (literally) in an uncaring environment. Doctors had little time to maintain connections to family, friends and their own health needs. Admitting fault, weakness or suicidality often resulted in medical board investigations.

Media restrictions on reporting doctor suicide lessen public awareness. In February 2019, a GP in regional Australia was found dead in a public park shortly before he was due to face court accused of filming and sexually assaulting his female patients. The media informed us there were 'no suspicious circumstances': they could not even say *suicide*. Nor are journalists emboldened to speculate why: shame, guilt, fear over his betrayal of his profession, family, and the terrible trauma inflicted on patients trusting their family physician.

Wible related the story of a medical student who deliberately walked in front of an Amtrak train in a very public death. His medical school said he died at home with his family. We agree with Wible that this type of self-censorship does nothing to prevent suicides in the medical sector. Euphemisms can't hide the truth of overdoses, hangings, shootings and jumping from hospital windows.

Physician suicide is complex. Doctors are different. They may have different personalities, their work is unique, and they are exposed to unusual situations. To suggest that doctors are more mentally unwell, have different brains or suicide genes in greater proportions than other White-collar professions is not supported by a shred of evidence. Their suicide is situation-based.

This phenomenon raises a question: why is it that we are so ready to pinpoint stress disorders among our soldiers in war zones and yet are so reluctant to even admit that there is occupational stress among doctors?

There is yet another professional category attracting attention. Durkheim wrote about suicide among the military some 122 years ago. Richard Holmes treated the topic in his *Acts of War* (1988). He discussed two escape mechanisms for those caught up in the Vietnam War: desertion and, more permenently, suicide. Rates were high, especially among the elitist soldiers and those who were retired. Military suicides are a major issue in the USA and now in Australia.

References

Hawton, K., Clements, A., Simkin, S., & Malmberg, A. (2000). Doctors who kill themselves: A study of the methods used for suicide. *QJM: An International Journal of Medicine, 93*(6), 351–357.

Homes, R. (1988). *Acts of war: The behavior of men in battle*. New York, NY: The Free Press.

Kay, A. (2017). *This is going to hurt* (pp. 106–107). London: Picador.

Kreimer, S. (2018). Preventing physician suicide: Recognizing symptoms, improving support suicide rate among docs. Is more than two times the overall population. *The American Association for Physician Leadership*. June 15. https://www.physicianleaders.org/news/-preventing-physician-suicide-recognizing-symptoms-improving-support.i.

Lieberman, H. (1976). *City of the dead*. Australia: Hutchinson.

Macdonald, K. M. (1995). *The sociology of the professions*. London: SAGE Publications.

Swannell, C. (2019a). Reducing risk of suicide in medical profession. *Medical Journal of Australia*, March 6.

Swannell, C. (2019b). Reducing risk of suicide in medical profession. *Medical Journal of Australia*. Published online: April 25, 2019. Sighted at https://www.mja.com.au/journal/2018/reducing-risk-suicide-medical-profession.

Turnbull, C. (1972). *The mountain people*. New York, NY: Simon & Schuster.

Wible, P. (2017). What I've learned from 1,103 doctor suicides. Posted on October 28, 2017 by Pamela Wible MD. Sighted at: www.idealmedicalcare.org/ive-learned-547-doctor-suicides/.

Chapter 13
The Alleviators

> *For me, an area of moral clarity is: you're in front of someone who's suffering and you have the tools at your disposal to alleviate that suffering or even eradicate it, and you act.*
>
> —Paul Farmer [American medical anthropologist and physician]
>
> *In every human being there is a wish to ameliorate his own condition.*
>
> —Thomas Macaulay [Thomas Babington Macaulay]

Abstract Presents ways of alleviating or deflecting suicide: by attracting a potential suicide to an ideology of some kind or engaging such a person in a 'belonging' activity like sport; and educating those who deal with self-death in critical suicide studies that look outside the conventional biomedical approach to the behaviour.

Keywords Belief · Belonging · Purpose in life

To alleviate is to lessen, soften or moderate a condition—like an ice pack on a burn, it relieves but doesn't cure. For some time we have been writing about alleviation of suicide rather than using the delusive word *prevention* (Tatz 2004). We also use the word in the sense of deflection, deferral and mitigation, that is, finding avenues that may give time for some reflection that may help delay a final act. Time out may still involve self-harm but it can stay the fatal exit. Some with suicidal thoughts have a shortened interruption period of self-destruction; others have prolonged or repeated periods. But our point is that any 'interruption' is a deflection.

We address two kinds of alleviation: first, social and physical programmes that engage persons, especially youth, that tackle loneliness, alienation, belongingness and perhaps inertia; second and separately, finding ways to rethink and reframe professional and public attitudes to self-death. The double-header is essential: there can be no success for the former if professional and public attitudes remain entombed

C. Tatz and S. Tatz, *The Sealed Box of Suicide*, https://doi.org/10.1007/978-3-030-28159-5_13

in concrete. The former are quintessentially simple, and the latter vastly complex and likely to take many decades of effort and resistance.

13.1   Ideology and Suicide

Ideology was once defined as the 'science of ideas'. Hardly that, ideology is nonetheless a collection of ideas and ideals, beliefs and values that have a political, social or religious purpose. The three Abrahamic religions are at once ideologies and ritualistic practices. ISIS or Islamic State or Daesh is a Salafi *jihadist* movement dedicated to a belief in the world supremacy of a Sunni Islamic world, the death or conversion of all infidels, and so on. It fires the faithful and converts the hapless and hopeless. Above all, it fuels belonging to a cause. Members have what psychiatrist Viktor Frankl called 'purpose in life'.

Many ideologies have led to nightmares, like both World Wars, and to the dozens of genocides in the last century. Irish poet William Butler Yeats published 'The Second Coming' in 1920 after viewing the ghastly wasteland left by European nationalisms: 'the ceremony of innocence' was drowned; the best lacked all conviction and the worst 'were full of passionate intensity'. The point in this context is that ideology arouses passion, and passion is a life force.

We don't know how many suicides or parasuicides have, or don't have, purpose. But it is a safe guess that a great many don't, either in a conscious or unconscious sense. Most suiciders don't leave notes of explanation, but those who do, often enough lament lack of hope or motivation, certainly any impetus to look forward or move forward with any sense of improved circumstances. Suicide is about the tenses, and the future variety isn't one of them.

Religious and political movements are tailor-made for purposefulness. Christianity offers the goal of a life hereafter; Hinduism, Buddhism, Jainism and Sikhism offer reincarnation. Communism in the twentieth century promised the redistribution of wealth. Any number of ethnic peoples has a driving conviction about sorcery and a spiritual world that controls destiny. Above all, these ideologies bring a sense of collectiveness, of not being alone, of averting alienation, of conformity and likemindedness rather than otherness. We may shudder at the surrender of free will and the succumbing to a mass, cultish movement but we can't deny the passionate belonging that is there for the believer.

We cannot imagine suicide prevention agencies proselytising in the manner of missionaries selling a particular story. But human inventiveness could put its minds to some form of ideology that envelops or rather inspires the 'patient' to want to belong. Malcolm X recognised that and he gave the fuel to fire Black Power, Black Islam in the 1960s and 1970s in America. The results weren't pretty, but he gave esteem and purpose to those who sorely lacked those qualities.

Belonging is also a matter of conformity, and we know that conformity is one of the most compelling forces in human society, at least amongst males. Holocaust historian Christopher Browning has given us a masterpiece in his book *Ordinary Men: Police Reserve Battalion 101 and the* Final Solution *in Poland* (1992). Some 500 men of varying ages and occupations, deemed unfit for the German army or the regular police, not Nazis, not indoctrinated, were assigned to guarding docks and warehouses in Hamburg, and then sent to the Lublin district of Poland. One evening in 1942, their commander, a regular soldier, told them tearfully that the next day they were to go to the village of Jozefow, round up all Jews, take them to the forest and there to shoot all, one bayonet length away from the back of their necks. If anyone did not want to do this, said Major Wilhelm von Trapp, step forward and be assigned other duties, without punishment. Nine stepped out. The rest went to Jozefow and then became the most efficient killing unit in that part of Poland, even inviting wives and girlfriends to spend weekends watching them 'at work'. Browning later interviewed a number of Battalion 101 members and one shocking conclusion emerged: they did it because they wanted to belong, to conform.

Dilemma: as with most things in life, there is good conformity and bad conformity.

Muscular Christianity was a philosophical movement that began in England in the mid-nineteenth century. It permeated the private school system with its cries for patriotic duty, manliness, militarism, the moral and physical beauty of athleticism, teamwork, discipline and self-sacrifice. To be effeminate was to be un-English. Muscular Judaism soon followed, in part to counter the premises and postulates of one Otto Weininger, an Austrian self-hating Jew, who depicted all things Jewish as 'feminine' and unworthy (Weininger 1903). (He killed himself at 23.)

Fads come and go, whether it be dancing the twist, twirling hula hoops, shaving one's head or other body modifications, like tattoos. But their hallmark is the collectivity: everybody is doing it and I can do it too, and I can belong. It is a passing alleviation of loneliness, alienation, inadequacy and anxiety. Fads don't have to await a creator, as in Barbie dolls: they can, with some thought, be imagined and then manufactured.

Modern music has at times encompassed elements of cultism, conformity and belonging. The 'Grateful Dead', the legendary San Francisco band (1965–1995), established a world-wide community of fans known as 'Dead Heads'. This close-knit fan base, identified by the wearing of iconic emblems and clothing, later initiated alcohol and drug support and suicide prevention campaigns. (Their keyboard player Vince Welnick slashed his throat in a shocking 'celebrity' suicide.)

Communism is passé, Boy Scouts is outmoded, nobody cares about Esperanto as a universal language, Christianity is 'boring', Black Power fits only one group, ISIS is often fatal and the Jonestown and Rajneesh cults are no longer. But there will always be a 'charismatic' figure somewhere, a cool messiah. In the words of poet W. B. Yeats: '… what rough beast … Slouches towards Bethlehem to be born?'

A tenable thesis lies in a relationship between suicide and political regimes that inspire admiration, perhaps security, and often enough, resistance. Russia, Lithuania, Latvia, Slovenia, Estonia and Hungary are in the top 10 high-rate suicide table. All admired or suffered Communism, and all appear 'lost' without the certain centrality that told them how to live, how to think, what to pray for. Israel is beset by enemies and has an outlook that is fuelled by a nationalism of resilience and resistance. South Africa, last on the suicide list, fought racial segregation and gross discrimination for close on three centuries and achieved freedom (of a kind) in 1994. It is too early to tell but there is every indication that now that the major triumph is there, suicide rates will rise.

A recent addition to suicide studies, Florian Huber's *Promise Me You'll Shoot Yourself: The Mass Suicide of Ordinary Germans in 1945* (2019), described how many Germans, brainwashed to fear the Bolshevik hordes, suicided *en masse* as the Soviet army invaded. With guns, poison, rope and water, entire families suicided, many, said Huber, from a sense of guilt or hopelessness, or seeing no other option after the defeat of their National Socialism ideology.

13.2   Sport and Suicide

We work in the world of sport history and find sport a fruitful avenue of alleviation, certainly of Aboriginal juvenile delinquency and, in all likelihood, suicidal behaviours.

An inspirational connection between sport and suicide is to be found in a fine work of non-fiction, H. G. Bissinger's *Friday Night Lights: A Town, a Team and a Dream*, published in 1990. (The television series was rated one of the best programmes of modern times.) A prize-winning reporter, Bissinger, spent a long time in the small rural city of Odessa in Texas. He chronicled the fortunes of the high school football team and the investment in it by the youth and the entire local population. The High School Panthers team was Odessa and Odessa was the Panthers, a symbiotic relationship vital to players and their devoted fans. Many sociological and psychological factors are involved here: physical space called 'home', my town and place, an external dynamic onto which could project, to which one can attach, wallow in, belong. Competitive sport has several components, one of which is the absolute essence—*not* knowing the outcome until the competition has ended. The future tense of sport makes sport what it is: once you know the result, a re-look at the video is but to watch an exhibition, not a competition. That future tense is highly significant for the would-be suicide: he or she wants to see out Friday night or Saturday afternoon.

The English novelist Nick Hornby put his finger on this point in an essay 'The agony of being a fan' (Hornby in Williams 1995):

Meanwhile, Neil Kaas will be watching his team lose to Brentford and Peterborough, red-faced with rage and frustration, and I'll be there when we go out of the Cup at home to Middlesbrough, say, or Manchester City. The quality of football will be poor (we know that already, most of us), the weather foul, the environment uncomfortable at best, intimidating at worst. There will be sweet moments for all of us, but they will be swamped by the sour … and we'll be happy, in our own peculiar way, saving up for a sunny day two or three years off in the future…

Yes, the sweet moments off in the future: that is the vitality and the lure of unpredictable sporting contests. The allure, even the despondency, is not in the past or even in the immediate present. So, is there evidence to support a connection between sport and reduced suicide? We need to stress that sport here doesn't simply mean the talent and the musculature to play. Sport is a broad church, with umpiring, judging, scoring, training, coaching, fund-raising, organising, recording, souvenir-making, selling and simple fandom all as much parts of the activity as the actual playing.

In Scottish soccer, the high and sometimes the low watermark is the passionate, often violent contest for supremacy between the Catholic team Celtic and the Protestant Rangers Football Club. They have played each other close to 415 times, with the matches won more or less equally. The passions are palpable—the sporting patriotism and the underlying religious fervour. Ideology and sport are conjoined. There is certainly a Ph.D. lurking there on the rates of suicide as between the soccer season and the off-season. There is a rough equivalent in Australian Rules football. There is a phrase, and a book, about one working-class suburb's team: *Kill for Collingwood* (Stremski 1986). The 'Magpies' seem intent on killing everyone else and the rest of the league reciprocates. And we do know that there is a 'dip' in the incidents and rates of suicide during the Super Bowl football finals in the USA. (On the other hand, domestic violence increases.) Another fruitful exercise would be to look at such relationships during World Series baseball and the Stanley Cup play-offs in North American ice hockey. Hornby's acute point is that even if one's precious team loses, there is always next season, next year, a reason to be there.

In English soccer, there is a tradition of spectator hooliganism (see Williams et al. 1984; Frosdick and Marsh 2018). The literature shows how important belonging and conformity go hand in hand among a group called the 'bovver boys'. [There is an enormous literature on how African–Americans felt when participating in race riots in the USA, especially in the events of Detroit and Los Angeles in the 1960s. Evidence showed that middle-class and professional people took part, not merely those that the one-time American Vice-President Spiro Agnew dismissed as 'riff-raff', blow-ins who were not part of the local scene.]

In 1895, Gustave Le Bon published *The Crowd: A Study of the Popular Mind*, a powerful work treasured by Hitler. In 1984, Bulgarian Nobel Laureate Elias Canetti published *Crowds and Power*. Both books analysed the difference between individual psyches and crowd psychology, the latter not just simply an aggregation of the individuals comprising it but a new, often monstrous force. A person can turn from being Dr. Jekyll to Mr. Hyde in specific settings.

There is no incontestable proof that the presence of sporting facilities and competition reduces the level of violence against the person, or general criminal or delinquent behaviour. But, at a level just short of empirical proof, there is no doubt that sports facilities, participation and competition have had a marked impact on 'junior' crimes against property and on assaults. Among dozens of examples, Port Lincoln in South Australia is a striking case: in winter, during the football season, juvenile offending by Aborigines is virtually nil. Off-season, it soars. Neither the police nor the Aboriginal community doubts the relationship. Other locales bear out both the assertion and the connection. The football season seems to lessen the level of vandalism, theft, graffiti and break-ins.

Art, dance and music may well be fruitful avenues of alleviation, distraction. Rock music in particular brings similar tribal affiliations and anticipations—the next album or tour, the motivation of social participation at concerts and festivals, the donning of emblematic clothing that identifies one as a fan; even the dangerous but enticing sharing of illicit substances bears similarities to sporting passions. One experiences the first rush of delight at a performance, and second and third watching or hearings heighten appreciation of the skills involved. In sport, it is the first match that evokes the *frisson*, that sudden high and low of expectation and hope. The team personifies the fan and the fans invest their souls in the team and its performances.

Colin Tatz's 1994 report (Tatz 1994), while raising the matter of suicide escalation in some detail, kept close to the relationship between sport and delinquency, which at that time had become a major concern. It concluded that:

- sport plays a more significant role in the lives of Aboriginal people than in any other sector of Australian society;

- sport provides a centrality, a sense of loyalty and cohesion that has replaced some of the 'lost' [tribal and ritualistic] structures in communities that so recently operated as Christian missions and government settlements;

- sport has become a vital force in the very survival of several communities now in danger of social disintegration;

- sport has helped reduce the considerable internalised violence—homicide, suicide, attempted suicide, rape, self-mutilation and serious assault—prevalent in some disordered communities;

- sport is a cheap enough option in the way it assists in reducing the second-highest cause of Aboriginal deaths, namely, from external and non-natural causes;

- sport has been effective in keeping youth out of serious (and mischievous) trouble during football and basketball seasons;

- sport has given several communities and regions an opportunity for some autonomy and sovereignty when they organise sport and culture carnivals;

- sport takes place despite the absence of facilities, equipment, money for travel, discrimination against teams and/or access to regular competition;

- sport in some regions takes place in circumstances and environs that often resemble the landscapes of Afghanistan in wartime and Somalia in drought time;

- sport is *essential* to counter the morale and moral despair of many Aboriginal people.

Harm and violence to property are not that far removed from harm to people. There is no concrete proof that they do belong in the same genre of behaviour. Nor is there ever likely to be such 'scientific' evidence. The best we can do is make reasonable and reasoned speculations, to work on what sociologist George Homans would call a high order proposition—in this case, just as sport appears to deflect delinquent behaviour of various kinds, so that activity will deflect, postpone or even deter suicidal thoughts or their completion. We go further and say that all the conclusions about sport and delinquency apply in the case of sport and suicide.

Several writers call sport one of the protective factors against suicide, but the connection has attracted remarkably little attention among suicide or sports scholars, particularly in Australia—a curious omission in one of the world's foremost sports-oriented societies. Apart from a brief mention of Australian football by McCoy (2007, 2008), no other author has mentioned, let alone considered, sport as part of that major agenda.[1]

There is some important evidence that there is a protective relationship. Sabo et al. (2005: 5–23) conducted a study of a representative sample of 16,000 US public and private high school students to see if there was a connection between athletic participation and suicide. There was a significant reduction in the odds of participants considering suicide among both males and females, as well as reduced odds of planning a suicide attempt among females in particular. With an admirable breadth of mind, the authors looked at classic sociological thought in the tradition of Durkheim. Their proposition was that being enmeshed in a social network of teammates, coaches, health professionals, community and family, the athletic participants experienced less anomie and a much greater sense of social integration. Moreover, they concluded, 'a commitment to organised sports gives adolescent participants something to lose' (Sabo et al. 2005: 5). The authors are keenly aware that sport promotes access and mobility for some groups, but that class, gender and race still preclude others, either historically or even contemporarily.

---

[1] To the best of our knowledge, only Curtin University in Western Australia has a student mental health programme that specifically encourages 'sport and recreation' and 'faith and religion' as protective activities.

Chioqueta and Stiles (2007: 375–90) studied 1,102 male military recruits, looking for the cognitive factors of engagement in sport and suicide risk. They found that 'students actively involved in sports exhibited less hopelessness'.

An even more compelling study by Babiss and Gangwisch (2009: 376–84) looked at sports participation as a protective factor against depression and suicidal ideation. Their findings are certainly encouraging. Sport, they stated, typically boosted self-esteem, improved body image, increased social support and had an impact on substance abuse. As sport participation increased, the odds of suffering from depression decreased by 25%, while the odds of having suicidal thoughts decreased by 12%. The study took into account sex, age, race, ethnicity, public assistance and physical limitations.

Brown and Blanton (2002) evaluated the relationship between physical activity, sports participation and suicidal behaviour among 4,728 college students in the USA. They found that sports participation was protective against suicidal behaviour: non-sporting men were 2.5 times more likely to report suicidal behaviour and non-sporting women 1.67 times more likely to do so. The Tomori and Zalor study (2000) is somewhat less helpful to that trend but remains another pointer. In a study of 4,504 secondary students, aged 14–19, 458 self-reported their suicide attempts. In that group, attitudes to sport were negative and their sport involvement was nil or negligible. This suggested that sport had some importance in the lives of the non-attempters, though the authors say they cannot claim that much about the relationship.

Curtis et al. (1986: 1–14) published a significant article on the 'dips' in suicide just before and during two important ceremonial sports events—the last days of the World Series baseball and the Super Bowl Sunday football event. Between 1972 and 1978, the suicide rates for the population were lower than normal on these specific days and higher thereafter; lower rates were also reported at the time of such public holidays as the Fourth of July and Thanksgiving. In essence, the study tested the Durkheimian propositions about the relationship between suicide and socially integrative activities—in this case, sport.

New Zealand has experimented with sport as a deflector. In 1997, the Aranui Sports Academy was established as a way of stopping the drift of Māori and Polynesian boys out of school (*North and South* 1997). Aranui High School switched from rugby league, at which they were champions, to rugby union in order to accommodate these young men. (The article does not explain why they switched codes.) In 1997, they beat St Bedes College in the final to win the schoolboys' championship. As the *North and South* magazine commented, such a predominantly Māori and Polynesian team victory would hardly arouse attention, but this was 'Christchurch, the most WASP-ish of all New Zealand cities and until this season, the final bastion of pre-Polynesian rugby'.

The organisers realised 'that one positive thing in many of these young people's lives was sport'. All 33 members of the Academy were properly enrolled in the school. The Academy's '*take* (purpose) is about changing the kids' attitudes in order to make them more employable, *not* about winning on the sports field'. Students had to complete four years of senior schooling or have been away from school for a year. In addition to sports activities, classroom work was compulsory. The boys set the agenda, 'no one else'. Needless to say, there was a howl of protest in Christchurch at the Academy's victory, with allegations of Aranui having brought in professional rugby union adults to demolish amateur children in union. The Aranui project could be emulated in any number of New South Wales towns, where the residential divide between East side and West side (as in Christchurch) is as great.

Building on the pioneering narrative therapy work of Michael and Cheryl White and New Zealander David Epston in the 1980s, David Denborough has been working with remote communities for many years. His book (2008), *Collective Narrative Practice: Responding to Individual Groups and Communities who have Experienced Trauma*, has an innovative chapter entitled 'The Team of Life: Offering Young People a Sporting Chance'. Sport, he contended, is a realm within which and through which life can develop richer meaning. It is indeed a glue that can hold a town or community together, as in Bissinger's study of Odessa. Sport not only provides lasting memories but enables 'young people who have experienced grave difficulties to speak differently about their lives'. The narrative therapy involves getting youth to answer what they like about a game, about creating a team of life, celebrating goals, tackling problems, avoiding obstacles and assisting others, whether in sport or beyond. Narrative therapy has developed as an effective process, especially in South Australia (Hunter and Milroy 2006: 151). It makes eminent sense to use metaphors and experiences that are known, are not threatening, give pleasure (albeit transiently), which do not involve what for many are the alien worlds of white coats, consulting rooms and heavy-duty pharmaceuticals. Plato, in Book III of his *Republic*, written some 2,400 years ago, told us that sport (gymnastics) was not just good for physical strength but for 'psychic harmony' and a way of avoiding doctors.

It is not unduly speculative to suggest that sport, especially the football codes, offers all young people in all cultures a mechanism for finding social meaning, 'a space of enjoyment and sociality', of not only being held or cradled but also of being held together. In the McCoy or Chandler–Lalonde analyses, it is a process of protection and of well-being. It is worth noting and regretting that much of suicidology tries to rest on an 'evidence-based' empiricism. One of the giants of modern sociology, Pitirim Sorokin (1889–1968), developed a remarkable theory of integralism, that is, that truth can be arrived at in three ways: through the senses, by reason and intuition, and through what anthropologists tend to call intuitive understanding or *verstehen* (Sorokin 1941). Our present preoccupation with methodology, especially mathematical methodology, often diverts us from both reason and *verstehen*—tools essential in this domain of explanatory difficulty.

Parker et al. (2006) introduced a programme of restoring and teaching traditional Aboriginal games into the communities of Cherbourg and Stradbroke Island in Queensland. The games are clearly culturally appropriate, holistic in several senses, and have been found to be acceptable as well as supportive of community well-being.

Kral's doctoral thesis (2009) reports a similar approach with a mix of scrabble, chess and ice hockey in Nunavut. In a personal communication (November 2009), he stated that a school in Nunavut established a racquetball team: 'The students loved it, the team did well against other community teams, and the suicides in their community stopped'.

There can be no debate about the role of sport in violent behaviour or of violent behaviour in sport. Violence is omnipresent—whether in chariot races in ancient Rome, or football matches in the UK from formal inception of the game, or in cricket riots in India, blood in the watersports at the 1956 Melbourne Olympics, the killing of 39 people at the infamous Heysel Stadium in Brussels in 1985, the football 'war' that erupted after the El Salvador versus Honduras match in 1969, attacks on Tour de France cyclists, the seemingly inevitable stoushes at ice hockey games, Mike Tyson biting off Evander Holyfield's ear in a 1997 heavyweight bout or serious physical clashes among Aborigines at Central Australian or Groote Eylandt football games. But sport, for the most part, is better at containing, dampening and restraining eruptions than most other activities.

The artificial enterprise we call sport provides what Durkheim deemed essential where there is a lack of true social coherence, namely, a truly collective activity, something that can fill the empty place within a life. For many young Aborigines, the emptiness is all too evident. They often live in places of despond, with little or no social distractions apart from video and game parlours. Many live inland, distant from the kind of fishing and food collecting that often diverts coastal people. Sport has a unique capacity to lay down rules and places of engagement, to codify its conduct and to spell out the sanctions that referees and umpires can administer. It can and does establish a body of lore, ritual, anecdote and mythology. It has the ability to become a cultural icon and a social institution; it can attract attention, gain adherents among players and supporters, and elicit loyalty across racial, caste and class barriers. It becomes what Durkeim, in 1897, saw as essential—an occupational group, a domain of meaningful social affiliation (Spangler 1979: 503), an avenue to what anthropologists Hugh Brody and Michael Kral called respect. It can help reconstruct, or at least imitate, a sense of kinship and reciprocity that once was. Sport fills lives that are meaningful and those that are empty. It is these qualities that give it such a significant role as a protector, perhaps even a prophylactic, against self-destruction.

13.3 Parliamentary Responses

Several parliamentary inquiries have been held in Australia: a Senate report in 2010, a House of Representatives investigation in 2011 and a number of state and territory investigations. All have a tone of lament in their titles: *The Hidden Toll* in the Senate report (Senate 2010), *Gone Too Soon* in the Northern Territory Legislative Assembly Report (2012).

Colin Tatz gave evidence to the Senate and Northern Territory Assembly committees, much of it on the lines of what has appeared in this chapter thus far. The Senate report made the expected recommendations: a national suicide register, better coronial reporting, more funding for prevention agencies and evaluation of them, improved training for all involved in suicide and mental health, training for those who are meant to assess at-risk persons. The Senate showed a great belief in setting targets for suicide reduction. It advocated support for research initiatives but said nothing about sport or similar activities. Witnesses and submitters of written statements came almost exclusively from persons in the mental health and prevention domains.

In many ways, the *Gone Too Soon* report was more direct, specific, more sharply focused on a number of issues. It wasn't as suffused as *Hidden Toll* on the mental health versions of suicide and in the end recommended that sport and recreation facilities be created at specified centres (Northern Territory Legislative Assembly 2012: xiii).

Music, dance and art are of the same genre when it comes to activities and mindsets that allow for focus on something else, that enables displacement of woes with thoughts and feelings of participation. Aboriginal youngsters with suicidal history have done well in 'purging' their frustrations through painting. In sum, these are activities that enable participation and participation usually, not always, leads to some understanding.

13.4 Bureaucratic Responses

A short paragraph: nil.

As discussed in our concluding chapter, the allocation of responsibility functions to departments and agencies is now so specialised that holistic approaches are nigh impossible. In a number of jurisdictions, one meets with the response that such and such is not their domain, try another one. Health says sport and recreation are not in their mission statements and sport says health is not their responsibility.

The simplicity of a research exercise is quite remarkable: there are several all-Aboriginal sports carnivals annually; there are any number of local support groups for a particular team in a small locale. Why not look at the suicide and parasuicide incidents in those places in a measure of time? Truly, not difficult and not expensive. But the biomedical model cannot unshackle itself from its visions, however ineffective they are in this field of human behaviour.

13.5   Critical Suicide Studies

The Critical Suicide Studies Network is a group of scholars from across the globe who have come together to establish a broader perspective of suicide. They have moved away from the constrained biomedical vision that pathologises distress and which obscures, and most often obviates, the social, political and historical contexts that contribute to that aspect of the human condition. Critical suicidology brings together academics, community activists, service users, practitioners, policy-makers, family members and persons with lived experience (White et al. 2015).

The transdisciplinary movement opposes the current one-size-fits-all evidence-based trend in suicide prevention/intervention in favour of collective and community-driven approaches. It takes a broader, wider perspective on suicide, unblinkered, unconstrained and not shackled by 'conventional wisdom' on suicide.

Critical suicide research works from the well-reasoned understanding that we need frameworks, strategies and concepts relevant for the complex, contemporary world in which we are now living or in which some are struggling for liveable lives. Diverse voices are welcomed. Research topics indicate the broader view of suicide: the times and regions of suicide; the choices people face; myths surrounding suicide; critiques of suicide 'gate-keeper' programmes; physician suicide; student suicide and athletes' suicide; autism and suicide; youth suicide; under-reporting of suicide and the reasons for that phenomenon; integrated prevention (or better, alleviation) programmes. The themes of this book, and the 'suicide notes' in the final chapter, are indicative of the network's approaches.

Suicide is enigmatic, puzzling and often enough incomprehensible. The critical suicide movement respects that: it explores the uncertainties, widens the contexts and, above all perhaps, challenges the dominant orthodoxies that have proven so unsuccessful.

References

Babiss, L., & Gangwisch, J. (2009). Sports participation as a protective factor against depression and suicidal ideation in adolescents as mediated by self-esteem and social support. *Journal of Developmental & Behavioral Pediatrics, 30*(5), 376–384.
Bissinger, H. G. (1990). *Friday night lights: A town, a team and a dream.* New York: Addison-Wesley.
Brown, D., & Blanton, C. (2002). Physical activity, sports participation, and suicidal behavior among college students. *Medicine and Science in Sports and Exercise, 34,* 1087–1096.
Browning, C. (1992). *Ordinary men: Police reserve battalion 101 and the 'final solution' in Poland.* New York: HarperCollins.
Canetti, E. ([1960] 1984). *Crowds and power.* New York: Farrer, Straus and Giroux.

Chandler, M., & Lalonde, C. (1998). Cultural continuity as a hedge against suicide. *Transcultural Psychiatry, 35,* 191–219.

Chioqueta, A., & Stiles, T. (2007). Cognitive factors, engagement in sport, and suicide risk. *Archives of Suicide Research, 11*(4), 375–390.

Curtis, J., Loy, J., & Karnilowicz, W. (1986). A comparison of suicide-dip effects of major sports events and civil holidays. *Sociology of Sport Journal, 3*(1), 1–14.

Denborough, D. (2008). *Collective narrative practice: Responding to individuals, groups and communities who have experienced trauma.* Adelaide: Dulwich Centre Publications.

Frosdick, S., & Marsh, P. (2018). *Football hooliganism* (2018 ed.). Uffcolme: Willan Publications.

Hornby, N. (1995). In G. Williams, *The agony of being a fan* (pp. 154–159).

Huber, F. (2019). *Promise me you'll shoot yourself: The mass suicide of ordinary Germans in 1945.* Melbourne: Text Publishing.

Hunter, E., & Milroy, H. (2006). Aboriginal and Torres Strait Islander suicide in context. *Archives of Suicide Research, 10,* 141–157.

Kral, M. (2009). *Transforming communities: Suicide, relatedness, and reclamation among Inuit of Nunavut, Canada* (Doctoral thesis). McGill University, Montreal.

Le Bon, G. (1895). *The crowd: A study of the popular mind.* New York: Dover Publications re-issue.

Legislative Assembly of the Northern Territory. (2012). *Gone too soon: A report into youth suicide in the northern territory.*

McCoy, B. (2007). Suicide and desert men: The power and protection of *kanyirninpa* (holding). *Australasian Psychiatry, 15*(S1), S63–S67.

McCoy, B. (2008). *Holding men: Kanyirninpa and the health of Aboriginal men.* Canberra: Aboriginal Studies Press.

North and South. (1997, October). East Side Story (pp. 74–80).

Parker, E., Meikeljohn, B., Patterson, C., Edwards, K., Preece, C., Shuter, P., et al. (2006). Our games our health: A cultural asset for promoting health in communities. *Health Promotion Journal of Australia, 17*(2), 103–108.

Sabo, D., Miller, K., Merrill, J., Farrell, M., & Barnes, G. (2005). High school athletic participation and adolescent suicide. *International Review for the Sociology of Sport, 40*(1), 5–23.

Senate Australia. (2010). *The hidden toll: Suicide in Australia.* Report of the Senate Community Affairs Reference Committee.

Sorokin, P. (1941). *The crisis of our age.* New York: Dutton.

Spangler, G. (1979). Suicide and social cohesion: Durkheim, Dreiser, Wharton, and London. *American Quarterly, 31*(4), 496–516 (Autumn).

Stremski, R. (1986). *Kill for Collingwood.* Sydney: Allen & Unwin.

Tatz, C. (1994). *Aborigines: Sport, violence and survival.* CRC Project 18/1989. Canberra: Criminology Research Council.

Tatz, C. (2004). Aboriginal, Maori and Inuit youth suicide: Avenues to alleviation? *Australian Aboriginal Studies,* (2), 15–25.

Tomori, M., & Zalor, B. (2000). Sport and physical activity as possible protective factors in relation to adolescent suicide attempts. *International Journal of Sport Psychology, 31*(3), 405–413.

Weininger, O. (1903). *Sex and character.* London: Heinemann.

White, J., Marsh, I., & Kral, M. (Eds.). (2015). *Critical suicidology: Transforming suicide research and prevention for the 21st century.* Vancouver: University of British Columbia Press.

Williams, G. (Ed.). (1995). *The Esquire book of sports writing.* London: Penguin Books.

Williams, J., Dunning, E., & Murphy, P. (1984). *Hooliganism abroad: The behaviour and control of English fans in continental Europe.* London: Routledge & Kegan Paul.

Chapter 14
Final Thoughts

Each victim of suicide gives his act a personal stamp which expresses his temperament, the special conditions in which he is involved, and which, consequently, cannot be explained by the social and general causes of the phenomenon.

—Émile Durkheim

Nothing in my life has ever made me want to commit suicide more than people's reaction to my trying to commit suicide.

—Emilie Autumn [American singer, song-writer and poet]

Abstract A set of concise reflections, speculations and suggestions on themes that are generally left out of the suicide discussion. Some matters are puzzling, some remain enigmatic, several resist solution, and a few offer some optimism. These notes encapsulate the essence of this book.

Keywords Suicide quandaries · Unresolved problems

Dwelling in dark domains, suicide (for most people) is best not talked about. But there is now some willingness to air the subject, especially as governments, prevention agencies and medical associations are bruiting 'mental illness', 'mental health' and setting (unattainable) targets for the reduction of these afflictions. Today, a coy readiness concedes the plight of the drought-stricken farmer, the terminal cancer patient, perhaps the bereft pensioner, certainly the overworked doctor. But legacies of the past—silence, shame, stigma, dogma, religious canon—block the paths to fresher thinking, possibly more effective thinking. We quoted Henry Miller in Chap. 1: what is new is often considered evil, dangerous, even subversive.

These notes on suicide may offer some clarity and some positive suggestions on aspects of suicide that are left out, sometimes ruled out, of the conventional box that walls off or walls in a behaviour that society rails against, gnashes teeth about, throws millions at, as the rates escalate and defeat us. What is involved here is not pessimism *versus* optimism, but realism.

14.1   Puzzles and Enigmas

14.1.1   'National Shame'?

A recent Australian tabloid headline cried out that the high rate of Aboriginal suicide was a 'national shame'. We understand the sentiment, but there is a serious misjudgement here. Certainly, the Australian nation and its component states and territories enacted legislation and introduced racist administrative practices that were draconian, each leaving its serious legacies on communities. There is shame in the national chronicle, but no state can ever be responsible for the decision of an individual to end a life, and no state can ever move successfully to a 'ban suicide' programme.

The esteemed pianist Hephzibah Menuhin turned sociologist. She once wrote that the greatest test of a nation's civilisation was the manner in which it treated its most underprivileged minority. Australia wouldn't score well on her rankings. The Aboriginal suicide rate is high and doesn't 'look good', but neither 'Australian-ness' nor 'Aboriginality' can be said to be a *causal* factor in suicide.

14.1.2   The Question of Rejection

Youth suicide is a particular anathema. Colin Pritchard, a British professor of psychiatric social work, suggested that suicide was a result of the suicider's ultimate rejection *by us*, our society (Pritchard 1995). We argue the polar opposite: it is not we who are rejecting the suicider but the suicider who is spurning us—rebuffing our love, family, our values, faiths, our creativity, our sense of hope and purpose, our life-saving and life-prolonging medical system, our imagination and, in a real sense, our whole civilisation. *That* is the ultimate affront and cause enough for our anger, our bewailing the numbers who take their lives, who seemingly kill themselves 'for no good reason' when there is so much on offer in life. A number of families have articulated the word 'affront' when challenging suicide verdicts of relatives.

14.1.3   Suicide and Other Deaths

Suicide scholars Crosby and Sacks (2002) contended that up to 400 people were exposed to any one suicide and at least 30 were significantly and negatively affected by each act of self-destruction. Unsurprisingly, there is a great deal of emotional reaction and a public grasping of any programme that helps to stop the behaviour.

People are momentarily attentive to a barrage of statistics about the numbers of young people who die on the roads each year. We tut-tut and mutter about raising the learner-driver age. We seem to be more accepting of young deaths by overdose, but are often judgmental about what is seen as an inevitable outcome for those who play around with illicit drugs or take 'ice' or ecstasy tablets for 'highs'. But suicide has a personal quality about it, an element of contempt for all that the collective *we*, the communal *us*, can offer. Barbagli would call much of this teenage suicide an act *against* us, society, the wider world. Our communal ego doesn't suffer that rejection with any grace. And those in the prevention business should consider how to address not nihilism but an antipathy to our offerings, our attractions to stay alive and participate.

Suicide ranks highly in causes of death in many countries: in Canada, New Zealand and the USA it ranks in the top ten, with Australia, the UK, France, Russia and Denmark not far behind. Drug overdose as a cause of death is quite high but is between 30 and 40 points lower than suicide. Road fatalities, measured in deaths per 100,000 of the population, show a relatively low rate in the UK, Denmark, France, Australia, climbing higher in Canada, the USA, with Russia remarkably high.

Overall, drugs, vehicle deaths and suicide loom large in all of these nations. But suicide is the issue that attracts the attention, the media, the battle cries for politicians. Accidents are viewed as inevitable; drug overdosing is regarded as somehow 'normal', yet it is suicide that creates a level of near-hysteria, a public outrage, something that warrants the label of scourge and 'curse'. Suicide is surely a public enemy.

Road deaths have been reduced through preventive measures—automobile technologies, improved roads and punitive measures for drink and drug driving. Suicide prevention has no such mechanisms, apart from rare cases such as gun restrictions or removing access to pesticides.

14.1.4 The Shroud of Taboo

Most people avoid talking, even reading, about incest, polygamy, cannibalism, eating dogs, female genital mutilation, priestly abuse of children, prison rape and venereal disease. But suicide stands alone when it comes to public discussion. One Australian example illustrates the matter.

Mindframe is an Australian government initiative aimed at encouraging 'responsible, accurate and sensitive representation of mental illness and suicide in the Australian mass media'. To minimise risk, media reporting should 'not glamorise suicide or provide specific details about the method or location of death'. These guidelines don't apply to senior school texts like Shakespeare's *Romeo and Juliet*, Tolstoy's *Anna Karenina*, Flaubert's *Madame Bovary* or to young audiences at Puccini's opera *Aida*, all of which end in suicide. Nor do they apply to one of the most popular television shows of all time, M*A*S*H, set in a field hospital during the Korean War (1950–1953), the last episode of which was the most watched programme in television history. The theme song, a Top 10 hit record, is titled 'Suicide is Painless'.

One should add that the 1993 novel by the American Jeffrey Eugenides, *The Virgin Suicides*, dealt with the self-killing of five adolescent sisters. Not only was it a popular novel, it also became a well-received movie—read and watched by hundreds of thousands. Nobody banned the book or the film because it showed all the details of how and why and when. 'Contagion', 'copycat', 'cluster suicide' were there for all to see.

Questioning media guidelines on suicide reporting invites a flurry of criticism. Copycat and cluster suicides are claimed to result from sensational and 'glamourous' reporting. No such guidelines apply to the reporting of rape, homicide, genocide, ethnic cleansing, terrorism, asylum-seeker boats capsizing and other barbarisms. What does a teenager make of a newspaper report that 'Rocky Rock Star' was found in a hotel room where 'there were no suspicious circumstances' or 'foul play is not suspected'?

Education departments, at least in Australia, don't allow talk of suicide for fear of giving youngsters 'ideas'. In Canada's Nunavut, the Inuit schools have corridors covered in notes from pupils who write down their suicidal thoughts, their calls for help, their desire to talk. Teachers and counsellors detect a correlation between openness and the amelioration of young deaths. Teachers are encouraged to give talks to students. Some American prevention agencies are now encouraging open discussions with secondary and tertiary students, adopting an inclusive approach. Given governmental blitzes on help for those with 'mental health issues', where and what is the purpose of taboo silence?

The taboo may no longer be a barrier to prevention activities, but the stoic silences are an obstacle to better understanding of suicide. Taking refuge in euphemisms may give families a fragment of solace. And since so many in any Western society are deemed 'mentally ill', there is comfort for the family of a suicider that their boy or girl was more or less 'normal'.

14.1.5   The Shroud of Stigma

The verb 'to commit' means, among other things, to perpetrate or complete something, most commonly, a scandal or a crime. We hardly ever say he or she suicided but rather *committed* suicide. The 'committed' here is remindful of the era when suicide was a sin, a crime in law, as in committing murder or treason. A stigma is a stain, a blemish and, above all, an unacceptable disfigurement of the soul of one's repute and standing. What the neighbours will think is a compelling social force, greater in some cultures than in others. In the end, it comes down to the simple word 'shame', a self-conscious emotion associated with negative feelings about the self. Shame is also related to guilt, real or imagined.

Prevention agencies often talk about getting rid of the stigma surrounding suicide. But neither they nor anyone else can eliminate an inherited cultural tradition, one steadfastly transmitted—osmosed perhaps—from one generation to the next. As we saw in Chap. 11, Andy Williams senior insisted he couldn't live with the verdict that Andy Williams junior had committed suicide: that he fell was possibly palatable, that he jumped was not.

14.1.6 The Matter of Sovereignty

We have talked about Foucault's ideas on biopower and biopolitics, that is, the mechanisms through which the basic biological features of the human species become the objects of a political strategy, of a general strategy of power. In short, Foucault's expressions meant government or state control, often enough through coercive power, of individual or population biology.

Foucault's concepts were pertinent in the context of suicide. The state exercises power over one's body in a range of ways—from birth control practices, compulsory sterilisation, to vaccination regimens, to prohibitions on circumcision laws on marriageable ages, multiple marriages, divorce, assisted dying and, as we have seen, suicide.

There is much debate in philosophy, law and biology about 'legal personhood'. Is a foetus a person? Does a foetus have rights? Is abortion an act of murder? What is a viable birth? Is personhood a matter of being, or having the capacity to function? In our context, the crux of the matter is who has sovereignty, autonomy, over one's anatomical, fleshly, human body? A biomedical and/or psychiatric view may well be that persons seriously defective or of diseased mind have no capacity to exercise that autonomy and therefore an agent/carer must make decisions for them, for example, whether a woman with a congenital disorder should be sterilised. That kind of decision usually rests, or should rest, with the natural parents or legal guardians. But history shows us that states intrude: biopower takes the form of legislation that makes the state the arbiter of reproductive capacity and leads to 'racial integrity acts' that sterilise a quite sentient and functioning Carrie Buck, discussed earlier. Noteworthy is that in 1920, the state of Tasmania set the tone for *Mental Deficiency Acts* that were to be enacted across the continent, many of them with eugenicist undertones.

By extension, we have seen the state intrude in the matter of suicide, criminalising, punishing, incarcerating those who thought they had the freedom to end their lives. By another extension, should the state seek to prevent self-cessation in the manner that it does? We readily agree that a suicide has serious impact on the families and friends of a suicider. But what interest does the wider society have in a private person's decision not to go on with life? There is no earthly evidence that a suicide is some kind of virus that affects a neighbour, a neighbourhood, a whole society. While there are, indeed, cluster suicides, as in some Aboriginal and Inuit communities, suicide per se is not a germ-like carrier of contagion.

Max Weber (1864–1920), the German sociologist and jurist, defined power as 'the ability of an individual or group to achieve their own goals or aims when others are trying to prevent them from realising them'. Their own goals: perhaps that is the essence of suicide—an exercise in sovereignty and in power, what Emanual Marx called 'the small seed of selfhood'? New Zealand academic Bering (2018) had a striking term for the action of someone stressed beyond endurance: *self-deliverance*.

14.1.7   The Antidepressant Puzzle

Articles in major newspapers, like the *New York Times* (30 November 2018), and in professional journals, have brought to the fore the relationship between suicide and antidepressant drugs. In one breath, so to speak, we have cries for the greater use of Ketamine, a drug used effectively in anaesthesia and which appears to work in cases of extreme suicidality, and warnings that the chemical has the opposite effect. We have material from an eminent Danish physician, Peter Grøtzche, that antidepressants lead to suicide, homicide and violent death (*British Medical Journal*, 3 September 2017).

So which is it? And indeed, is it an either/or? The high road of biological psychiatry and more pharma therapies that do work for some people; or the low road of what we might call 'social psychiatry'—the network of factors that lie outside the immediacy of the synapses and inside Durkheim's 'social conditions'? Medical practitioners, equipped with a limited toolkit, reach for the prescription pad too readily—perhaps because the social conditions of their patients are too insurmountable or lie too far beyond their scope of practice; or there are simply few other medical alternatives available and patients want *something* to alleviate their ills.

14.1.8   The Statistical Puzzle

The quote below is taken from 'Figures in Mental Health', located on the website of the Black Dog Institute, an Australian agency devoted to matters of depression and anxiety states:

> Mental illness is very common. One in five (20%) Australians aged 16–85 experience a mental illness in any year. The most common mental illnesses are depression, anxiety and

substance use disorder. These three types of mental illnesses often occur in combination. For example, a person with an anxiety disorder could also develop depression, or a person with depression might misuse alcohol or other drugs, in an effort to self-medicate. Of the 20% of Australians with a mental illness in any one year, 11.5% have one disorder and 8.5% have two or more disorders. Almost half (45%) Australians will experience a mental illness in their lifetime.

The census population in Australia in 2016 was 24.1 million. In that year, urinary disease, flu and prostate cancer each took some 3,300 lives. The suicide figure was 2,866. Given that some 4.8 million people were deemed as having a mental disorder that year, and since disorder is said (not proved) to be the basis of all or most suicides, how can we explain that only 0.04% of the 'disordered' suicided? What of the remaining 99.96%, or any other proportion of that cohort, and their depression? Were they prevented from taking their lives through the suicide prevention campaigns and medical interventions, or is depression nothing like the foundation on which suicide is said to rest? The figure of 0.04% self-deaths among the 'mentally ill' hardly warrants the hysteria that surrounds suicide. And who, indeed, gets agitated, let alone messianic, about urinary deaths?

14.1.9   The Pain Puzzle

Our view is that most people would say that assisted dying to end unendurable physical pain is understandable—even when they disapprove of such a manner of death. Yet the same people cannot, or say they cannot, condone the dying of the suicider with excruciating psychache, the acute mental pain. Why is that?

14.1.10   The Medical Bias Puzzle

One needs to ask why it is that when a youth suicides, particularly an Aboriginal youth, the instant response is that this must be occasioned by mental illness. But when a doctor or psychiatrist takes their life, we are met with long explanations that have little to do with mental illness: long hours, stress, burn-outs, bullying and harassment, dealing with others' illness takes its toll, the constant worry of litigation and malpractice, a health system that promotes profit and 'throughput' over considered, personal care and fear of failure. One explanation provides situational context, and the other leaps to labels.

14.2   The Biomedical Model

14.2.1   The Medical Obsession

The century of obsession with mental illness and mental wellness has confined suicide into a neat box that brooks few further insights or investigations into causation and explanation. The medical paradigm has an inbuilt distortion. Medicine operates best on empirical evidence. It likes hard and sharp edges—visible, documentable, replicable qualities and evidence-based trials that lead to the most effective therapies and treatments. The scans, screenings and pathology tests become best practice. Modern medicine disdains 'alternative' treatments: homeopaths, naturopaths, chiropractors and the like are regarded as quackery, pseudo-health care without any *evidence*. Suicide is regarded as a medical matter, but there are no sharp or even blunt edges to be detected in the way that most illnesses present. Alternatives are given glancing consideration. The end result is that we label as 'disorders' as many behaviours as possible—in the hope that one can capture an edge, a hook on which to 'contain the epidemic', to pin a therapy.

The Durkheim quote at the start of this chapter is crucial to the whole suicide 'problem'. Each act of suicide is directly related to two things: the temperament or personality of the suicider and the 'special conditions' in which they are involved. Personality means character, individuality, disposition, with an enormous range of qualities—from surly and reticent to carefree and outgoing, from gregarious to reclusive, from dull to charming, from inwardness to expansiveness, from thin-skinned to accommodating. The conditions range from wealth to poverty, from safety to insecurity, from inclusion to exclusion, from violence to harmony. Sociologists and anthropologists are better trained to look at such conditions than medical people. Specialists who devote their lives to lungs, hearts, kidneys and livers focus not on personality or temperament; on the operating table or viewed through a scan, these characteristics are irrelevant. Psychologists are versed in matters of personality and rarely in conditions of life (despite the A\$14 million a week spent on their services in this country.) Yet social science, said Durkheim, generally cannot explain the relationship of each of these factors to a suicide—and nor can medicine. But if nearly all behaviours and emotional states are 'disorders' (as the *DSM* tells us), then one can deem everything as somehow definable, perhaps containable, namely, 'a mental health issue'.

14.2.2 DSM *and Children's Suicide*

Until recent times, suicide statistics reported the youngest as the 14 or 15–24 bracket. Suicide of those under 14 was rarely presented, partly in the belief that it never occurred. That has changed. An article by Hanna in a CNN report in 2017 lamented that in the USA between 1999 and 2015, 1,309 children between 5 and 12 took their own lives.

Child suicide in England was addressed by William Ireland in his major book—*The Mental Affections of Children*—published in 1898. By 1870, public education for children became the law in England and that was what Ireland investigated—imbecility and insanity. But while he dealt with such affections [pathologies], he found that the major cause of child suicide was an external agency—'being punished or harshly treated by their parents or teachers'.

By contrast, the *DSM* brooks no such discussion of outside agencies in child suicide. Instead, this 'bible of psychiatry' asserts that child suicide is attributable to any one of 13 mental disorders—ranging from ADHD to schizoaffective disorder, depressive disorders, disruptive mood dysregulation disorder, separation anxiety disorder, to oppositional defiant disorder. It would seem that parents, teachers, classmates, the playground or cyber gadgetry are not related in any way to these early self-inflicted deaths.

14.2.3 The Question of Rationality

Earlier, in Chap. 2, we quoted psychiatrist Norman Kreitman as doubting the very existence of rational suicide. Immanual Kant (1724–1804), a philosopher of the highest standing, was against suicide and believed it was not the act of a rational person. Yet he conceded that in some circumstances, one must be prepared to surrender life and 'not disgrace the dignity of humanity' (Battin 2015: 425). The Dutch philosopher Baruch Spinoza (1632–1677) argued that reason demanded that every person should love his or her self: therefore, suicide was an illogical act (Battin 2015: 303). Spinoza was a deeply religious man, and his dictates raise another question: can one argue that religious people see suicide as irrational or unreasonable while non-believers perceive a clearer division between reason and unreason? There is not much research on religious affiliation and suicide, but one major essay by Dervic et al. (2004) is pretty typical: the researchers do their work among patients diagnosed with depression. It would be good to know whether non-depressive atheists are less or more inclined to suicide than non-depressive believers, that is, unless you start with the premise that the only people who take their lives are depressives.

'In some circumstances' was Kant's way of saying it; 'special conditions' was Durkheim's phrasing. We have traversed a number of these situations in this book, and they all add up to the sense of suicide in the face of impossible or seemingly impossible choices. There are, indeed, times when death by one's own hand is the most sensible escape mechanism. Rationality here means a wilful, sentient, conscious state of mind by a person capable of forming an intent. It is much easier and more convenient to view suicide as irrational.

There is always a tension between the way law and medicine view rationality. The legal view tends to focus on sentience—which is the ability to perceive one's environment and experience sensations such as pain and suffering, or pleasure and comfort. The medical view is fuzzier. It starts with the premise that many in a population suffer a disorder of some kind, and once that base theory comes into play, so does the notion that a disorder either interferes with rationality/sentience or impairs that faculty. One has only to look at the conflicts that occur daily in courts to see how the legal and the medical perceptions diverge.

14.2.4   The Matter of 'Happiness'

The other distortion, of course, is that wellness is happiness and the absence of that quality means sickness and that, too, must be medically rather than socially addressed. We have said that many of the suicides—among the 36 categories presented in Chap. 6—arise from the social order. Choosing to die for shame, dishonour, country, a cause, religion, or a cult has nothing whatever to do with happiness or wellness, disorder, unwellness, and no therapies are warranted, let alone to hand. Oh, we don't mean *that kind of suicide* is a response one often hears. And if not *that* kind, then what kind do the professionals and the preventionists have in mind?

In the West, we persist with the happiness–wellness myth, that we are born with a human right to be 'happy' and any diminution of that quality necessitates treatment. Viktor Frankl, among others, has presented us with a precept that we instantly reject: that to live is to suffer. We all 'suffer the slings and arrows of outrageous fortune', as Shakespeare wrote. We endure a range of hurts: pain, betrayal, loss, discrimination, disappointment, frustration, impotence, poverty, hunger, dislocation, insecurity, ailment, affliction, alienation, invasion, war, bureaucratic blunder, accidents, retrenchment, ostracism, rejection, failure. Anxiety is hardly a visitation from outer space, and anxiety is, wrongly in our view, too often equated with depression and/or unwellness. We live on a planet beset by suffering, from daily murders, rapes and assaults, to earthquakes and tsunamis that destroy hundreds or thousands, to devastating climate change floods and fires, to ethnic cleansings and genocides, to droughts and famines, to civil and uncivil wars, to 60 million refugees seeking shelter of some kind. 'Happiness' is best manufactured in Hollywood's dream factories.

14.2.5 The 'Oneness' of Suicide

We have presented 36 categories of suicide, many of them with different motives and occurring in divergent social and political contexts. There may be more. One can think of many deaths which could fall into a category called '*situational suicide*', the result of a whole chain of events. The 'suicide problem' needs to be seen as many-sided, some as addressable where an intervention can stop a young person who, unable to see around the corner or lacking the resilience to cope, acts impulsively; many as unfathomable, some scarcely preventable.

While suicide is suicide, there is a world of difference between a teenage *jihadist* bomber brainwashed or coerced into 'martyrdom' by killing others, the bankrupt who doesn't wish to face ignominy, the farmer who despairs of ever seeing rain, the addict who seeks only oblivion, the Armenian woman faced with what she perceived as impossible choices, the person who is jammed between a rock and a hard place, the right Juliets who have fallen in love with the wrong Romeos.

As with the wars on cancer or on drugs, the failure, perhaps the refusal, to distinguish categories or sub-species of the target dooms the chances of 'victory'. Once one is prepared to see the differences in 'types', one is forced to recognise that there are causal factors that lie in contexts other than 'the disturbed mind', that there are cogent and rational reasons for wanting to cease, and that a predestined 'suicide gene' is not responsible for risk-taking or for dicing with death in many circumstances. Suicide, as the eloquent French physician Esquirol told us way back in 1845, is not a disease.

Mental health is a convenient toolbox. That container has borders, perimeters and parameters and allows for a [false] sense of control of the matter. Suicide as mental illness narrows the causation problem and infers that prevention is always possible. External factors, what Durkheim called 'special conditions', are too numerous, too complex to comprehend, let alone to treat. The question comes down to this: do those who deal with suicide not know how to approach external factors, or is it that they don't want to?

As humans, we all need support and assistance in making social decisions. Reproduction is but one reason for marriage or cohabitation: having someone to share or discuss decision-making is another, even in male-dominating cultures. In the latter, the social assistance comes from male relatives, and if not fathers then uncles who figure largely in their lives. The loss of that kind of internal support, or the feeling that it is lost, often enough causes withdrawal from family and then from society—withdrawal, in the sense of no longer caring about participation as a member of society. That, wrote anthropologist Emanuel Marx, was the social context of violent behaviour, and that was what makes suicide the flipside of homicide (Marx 1976). What he was contending was that violence of either kind arises out of the social order, not the realm of mental disorder. It also leaves one pondering why we believe we can prevent suicide but not homicide?

There is an interesting duality in medico-legal attitudes to murder and to suicide. In homicide, the thrust of defence lawyers is to seek mitigation, even exculpation, by virtue of mental illness, while prosecutors do their best to exclude such a defence, seeking conviction and punishment of what they see is a criminal, wilful, rational act. Yet in suicide, all involved seem bent on finding mental illness as the explanation, and exculpation in as many cases as possible. Thus, the murderer who takes a life is bad and the suicider who takes a life is mad.

This duality goes further: not too long ago, most Western legal systems regarded drunkenness not as an excuse but a mitigating factor in sentencing a driver for, say, manslaughter. The logic of the MacNaughten Rules was that a person in such a mental state had no intent and may not, at accident time, have been conscious of the wrongness of the action in question. In later years, drug or alcohol presence exacerbated the offence and the punishment was harsher. But 'mental illness' or 'disorder' makes it all softer.

14.2.6   Good Grief, Bad Grief

The now old-fashioned *melancholy* was once believed to derive from the four humours: blood, phlegm, yellow bile and black bile. Immense sadness was the hallmark of melancholy, and sadness was inevitably associated with loss of some kind. Everyone suffers loss at some point: ambitions that are thwarted, status that is diminished, comfort that becomes discomfort, a parent or child who dies, decreased mobility, unreliable memory. As Johann Hari has said, we lose connections and the loss is grief—internal sadness, torment, anguish. Grief has any number of dimensions: physical, cultural, spiritual, social, cognitive. Suicide is but one escape mechanism.

Melancholy, sadness, grief are part of the normal nature of things, not manifestations of disorder. A number of psychiatrists contend strongly that prolonged grief is a mental disorder (PGD) and should be listed in the *DSM*. Long before psychiatry was born, most societies and cultures had well-defined mourning rituals that learned how to deal with prolonged grief. Trained grief counsellors are not thick on the ground. They ought to be. Given that we live in an age where we are told, often cajoled, to 'move on', we need tutoring in how exactly we can move on from loss—without resorting to suicide or some other form of self-harm. Pills can't do that.

14.2.7   Assisted Dying

The Western world is ageing, with much higher life expectancy rates than a few decades ago. Several countries have male–female average ages over 80: Japan 83.7, Switzerland 83.4, Singapore 83.1, Australia 82.8, USA 79.3. Several African countries have an age expectancy of 49. Longer life ensures problems of aged care, of personnel, institutions, equipment, costs. And while prolongation is the dedicated aim of all those involved, some people simply don't want to continue.

As of March 2018, only eight countries, eight American states and Australia's state of Victoria have legalised assisted dying. Faced with legions of people who need care, often constant care, people who have little quality of life, some who don't even know that they are alive, the reluctance to legalise this kind of elected death is unfathomable. One has to question how realistic is the mantra that such death is a 'slippery slope' going down to the Nazi era, to greedy relatives who can't wait to get their hands on the loot, to those who 'want to get away with murder'.

The safeguards and roadblocks in current legislation would certainly preclude the homicidal relatives from acting in haste and unobserved. Before one leaps to opposition to assisted dying, a deeper look at the history books will spell out the enormous differences between Nazi biopower and its bureaucratic procedures and the present-day qualifications required by today's requester of such a form of exit.

In this book, we have questioned the whole modern suicide paradigm. We also question the basis of medicine's holy grail of prolonging life no matter the circumstances. There are persons who want to die, 'to cease upon the midnight with no pain'; there are those who need to die, to put an end to humiliation, dysfunction, helplessness, pain, and in Viktor Frankl's language, there are those who no longer have any purpose in life.

14.3 Prevention Problems

14.3.1 The Preventable and the Non-preventable

If stopping suicide is the societal goal, then agencies and their funders need to articulate and then target those who can possibly be deflected from self-death and those who cannot be, by the nature of their motive or circumstance.

Suicide preventionists mislead with their 'zero target' obsessions. Prevention is aimed at the vulnerable. The teenager struggling, the youth who sees no hope, the 30-something male separated, alone, adrift from children and family, the financially ruined, the lonely—they are the 'at-risk' people where suicide prevention has some 'success'.

There can be no overt markers or bleepers for those who feel shame, dishonour, guilt, obsessive loyalty to a cult or social or political movement or a leader, or who suffer pervasive hopelessness. Nor can there be an intervention in those who flirt with, even invite, acutely dangerous behaviour. Unless the preventionists can pinpoint, however broadly, the cohorts they are aiming at, their efforts will continue to fail.

There is also the matter of what prevention means, or is meant to mean. It can never mean eliminating the action, as with smallpox. It can mean deflection to another path, deferral for a period of reconsideration, alleviation of some conditions, symptoms or pain that are immediately overwhelming. It can mean respite in all its senses. It can mean sedation in pharmaceutical modes, or sunlight in a sanatorium, not a psychiatric ward.

14.3.2 *The Target Fantasy*

Suicide Prevention Australia (SPA) is a major body in this field. In 2016, it advertised a tourist trek though the Larapinta Aboriginal tribal lands in the Northern Territory. The slogan was 'Hike to Halve Suicides'. Hyperbole, certainly, and hardly big money, but it indicated a mainstream belief in a money solution. Since then, the major political parties have been agitating about targets and formulating policies to set them and achieve them.

At the same time, SPA called for strong action by government 'to contribute to our shared goal of halving suicide in ten years' (media release, 8 June 2016). Such idealistic phrasing leads agencies into a self-defeating position because they, too, base their strategies on the flawed, traditional, 'official' *rates* of suicide. Rates are increasing because more people in the mainstream population are taking their lives; because population numbers have swelled by intakes (and often harsh detention) of severely distressed migrants, refugees and asylum-seekers; because sexual violence soars; because toxic prescription drugs proliferate and opioids abound; because younger and younger children are given potentially toxic medications; because 'ice' and ecstasy become cooler; and because coronial practices are now more willing to determine suicides than hitherto. And coroners now have a lower burden of proof to work on. The Tollefsen study (2012) of suicide statistical reliability showed something of the gap, even the gulf, between actual suicides and officially determined suicides. In many countries, the suggestion is that reality is twice the official rate. Prevention strategies might have greater success if they promoted and promised more realistic outcomes, like differentiating suicide by categories, by addressing very specific age, geographic, religious or ethnic groups, by improving 'suicide-at-risk' surveys and aftercare of hospitalised patients, rather than chasing an ever-moving target, a chimerical 'halving of rates'.

Why do preventionists persist in believing that more of the same is better than the same? Will more money, more websites, more warnings before Netflix dramas or restrictions on media reports of celebrity suicide, more asking 'R U OK?' somehow achieve what has eluded the mental health sector for a hundred years? The reality is that more of the same isn't reducing suicide and is hardly likely to.

In Chap. 4, we discussed the ferocity with which the Renaissance and Enlightenment eras attacked suicide and those who attempted it. Today, we have democratic governments proclaiming war on suicide, pledging 'elimination', agencies dedicated to 'halving' the incidence, many of them with a similar ferocity. Do we ever stop to question why, as Montesquieu did in 1721? Why would you want to stop someone ending an unendurable existence of physical or mental pain even when you know you can't cure it, alleviate it, palliate it? 'Suffer it', or God's will, are common answers, astonishing responses in an age where billions are spent on chemicals and psychological services to stop suffering.

14.3.3 Holism: Preventionism and the Public

Apart from his presidency of the Bell Telephone Company, the American Chester Barnard (1886–1961) was renowned as a leader in the fields of public administration and organisation studies. He always maintained that the success of any organisation depended on the manner in which it saw, and included, the clientele being served to be a partner in the organisation whole, a sector as important as the executive and the staff (Barnard 1949). Following his dictate, we argue that the medical and nursing professionals, the suicide researchers and the preventionists need to embrace the general public in their operations and findings. In short, the more that suicide discussion is opened up and not confined to the 'mental illness industry', the more prospect there is of some amelioration of the prevalence of suicide.

The lack of inclusion of many Aboriginal communities has led to an insistence, at least in some regions, that suicide is their problem and only they can solve it. Community 'ownership' has its merits and achievements, but 'going it alone' is not always the effective answer. If ever there was need of Barnard's partnership, of a two-way involvement, then it lies in suicide amelioration.

14.3.4 The Allocation of Functions

Holism requires a generalist frame of mind, an ability to embrace broad perspectives to multi-factorial agendas. Specialisation leads to great refinements and results. But some matters, like suicide, need all the help they can get. In the past century, specialist departments of government (and universities) replaced generalist units to the point where jurisdictions border on the absurd. A limb surgery practice in a Sydney professional suite has signs indicating left for above the elbow, below the elbow, below the wrist, right for above the knee and below the ankle. Suicide is not treatable, let alone by the digits.

Government agencies are leaning in that direction. When you mention sport to a state health department, their answer is 'go to the sports department, that isn't our domain', and vice versa. Lateral thinking isn't a virtue of specialisation. A dedicated 'suicide commission' bringing specialists together under a generalist could well produce better outcomes in reducing or alleviating suicide.

14.3.5 The Allocation of Personnel

In 1969, Laurence Peter and Raymond Hull published what they thought was a satirical book on management, *The Peter Principle*. Soon enough they found they were describing the reality of the principle: 'that in a hierarchy everyone rises to their own level of incompetence'. One may succeed in previous jobs, but then one hits a wall which indicates that one doesn't have the wit or the skills to go any further—and incompetence rules.

There are many, too many, in the field of suicide who don't reach their incompetence level: they are inept from the start—*sans* training, *sans* formal education, mentoring, even apprenticeship in its broadest sense. Harsh that may sound, but what other branches of medicine, or any profession, entrusts suicide diagnoses (where possible), treatments (where possible) and prevention (nigh impossible) to persons with either no formal tuition, or less than an hour's exposure in undergraduate curricula, moreover, persons with zero education in disciplines that have something to tell us about suicide.

In what other field of sensitivity such as suicide do we find legions of volunteers offering their services to 'prevent' a person wanting an exit? Suicide is, after all, an amalgam of history, geography, environ, context, family, ability and disability, illness and wellness, employment, income, access to social assistance, loneliness, alienation.

The *raison d'etre* of 'doing good works' is admirable, but if good works are to achieve any goals, they need enough training to recognise their levels of capacity.

14.3.6 The Distribution of Personnel

Allowing for the moment that only psychiatrists, and perhaps doctors, are the professionals who can, and should, deal with suicide, one has to ask questions about their distribution across the Australian population. We have not looked at this factor in other nations. Some 67% of Australians live in eight cities, the remaining 33% mainly in rural areas and some 500,000 in remote locations. The distribution of GPs per 100,000 of the population is stark: 101.3 for urban areas, 71.3 for remote regions and 61.5 for very remote locations (RACGP 2018). The distribution of psychiatrists is even bleaker: some 88% practise in urban centres. The general attitude towards those in non-urban settings is 'well, try private practices'—of which there are less than a handful.

In a land of enormous distances, and of costly small airline fares, in a land of chronic drought and daily heat, the remote ones need as much succour as they can get. Priests may be passé, but practitioners of medicine and pill-prescribers are not.

14.4 Non-medical Approaches

14.4.1 The Social Sciences

Suicidology is not a science; however, much statistical comparisons and analyses give it such an appearance. Most suicide studies are based solely on official rates of deaths per 100,000 of the population, reliant on that kind of available arithmetic. We have discussed the problems of coronial practice and will refer to them again below. Here, it needs to be said that decimal points, regression analyses and chi-square correlations give little insight and offer no solutions to the behaviour.

History is as good a starting point as any in trying to understand suicide in society. We need to note cultural, political and religious practices, insights and attitudes, particularly in multicultural states. We also need sociological and anthropological approaches: fieldwork, a much heavier reliance on informants, visits to locales, checking with documents where possible, a willingness to listen to anecdotal evidence (without the implied condemnation that anecdotes are always suspicious or dubious), and a fair degree of participant observation, using what the German language calls *verstehen*, or intuitive understanding. Suicide cannot be subjected to double-blind and control tests as with many diseases and their therapies. Often enough, a 'feel' for what's happening is a far better litmus than a microscope.

Suicide is an 'inside' phenomenon, and if amelioration or intervention is to be needed, then the closer the observer or therapist is to the person or to his or her environ the better. The conditions and context can be talked about in a consulting room, but not experienced by the consultant.

Suicide is an interior–exterior phenomenon, at once internal to the body and mind of the one contemplating the action, and that person located in a milieu of some kind.

The internal and external dynamics differ between persons, even those in the same familial group. Hence the need of preventionists to address prospective suicides in differing ways. There is never going to be a one magic bullet solution, one pill, one injection.

14.4.2   Anthropology in Particular

We contend that an anthropological lens is the most likely discipline to produce an understanding rather than an explanation of why a person has ended life. In many countries, and certainly in Australia, there is a coronial or medical examiner head office which is informed of suspicious deaths by way of summary sheets supplied by the police service located in the deceased's place of death. That is where depositions—that is, witness's sworn out-of-court testimonies—are taken. This is a process of gathering information as part of the discovery process and, in some circumstances, may be used at inquests. For those delving into a particular suicide or suicide generally, it is these locales that will provide insights from teachers, nurses, doctors, scout masters, priests, pharmacists, police, counsellors, lawyers, ambulance personnel, sports trainers, social workers, liaison officers and, of course, kinsfolk. A forensic anthropologist has the skill to synthesise such collected materials. Therein is the archive of the suicide's life and death, not in the coroner's head office, not in a statistics bureau. The depositions will reveal whether or not there is any evidence of mental illness or signs that could or should have been noted. [Colin Tatz used such depositions for his Aboriginal suicide study in the 1990s; those files had not one mention of 'mental illness' in 43 Aboriginal suicides in 14 rural New South Wales towns in a two-year period.]

In sum, quality suicide research needs legwork and fieldwork: paperwork is not good enough if one is investigating the contexts of individual or even cluster deaths.

14.5   Courses of Action

14.5.1   Recognising the Violence Syndrome

Ambiguity is a tactic long used by governments. Blurred lines of responsibility, unclear accountability and channels of communication, deflection of demands by real or imagined crises leave one in a state of uncertainty, off balance. In this way, governments have some control over crises and can juggle competing demands and grievances. Election time is a good place to look at ambiguity: lower taxes, higher taxes, investigating the treatment of the disabled, aged care, paedophile priests, the behaviour of banks, higher wages, more jobs, more coal, less coal, power prices, increased aid to church schools, free abortions and so on.

Aboriginal Australians suffer more ambiguity than most people: citizens, not citizens, equal, not equal, humans and then Others. There is, as shown elsewhere, a link between ambiguity and patterns of behaviour. A syndrome comes into play. First, *frustration*, followed by a sense of *alienation* from society, of not belonging; then *withdrawal* from society, no longer caring about membership, loyalty or law-abiding behaviour; and then the threat of, or actual, *violence.* That violence is either towards others or towards self. Here, we see Barbagli's *for* and *against* suicide played out.

The syndrome isn't confined to Aboriginal youth, but in their case the ambiguity and violence syndrome are starkest. Apart from an intelligent counsellor in a one-on-one set of meetings, how can one possibly track these stages in a context of ambiguity?

14.5.2 'The Knowledge'

Before the advent of Global Positioning System (GPS), all London cab drivers had to achieve and pass 'the knowledge', their licence to provide a service in that city. When one walks into a consulting room of a dentist, surgeon, physician or vet, one is confronted by an array of framed certificates telling us that the '-ologist' we are calling upon is duly trained, fully certified, and registered to practise that profession. They have the knowledge. We are gladdened by the fact that the professional has been examined and passed fit. The reassurance of professionalism is there before you enter the sanctum.

Apart from a handful, perhaps two handfuls, of suicide scholars in Australia, usually in academic positions, what certificates are possessed by those who engage clinically with potential suiciders? Two decades ago Colin Tatz was asked to join three psychiatrists in presenting material to 40 psychiatry registrars from two Sydney universities: they wanted the quartet to give a two-day live-in seminar on suicide—because, they claimed, they had no formal training or education on the external factors involved in suicide and needed it for practice.

Little has changed. Suicide always comes under the rubric of 'mental health' and that, too, is given limited time. At present, even mental health has been dropped in the training regime of mental health nurses in Australia. So, with an alleged one in five or even one in three of the population suffering 'mental illness' or 'disorder' and since 'disorder' is seen as the *sine qua non* of suicide, what is it that we are doing? In all other branches of medicine, would we license a practitioner to carry out surgery, or nuclear radiology, or renal care with so little tuition?

The lack of formal training for the many who engage in the suicide phenomenon is quite staggering. It is also ludicrous given the attention and money devoted to the matter. More than 150 projects and strategies operate for Australia's now 25 million population. That involves a large number of workers and volunteers. Given the history and the sociology of suicide, and its increase each year, one has to ask how equipped the personnel are to deal with this behaviour. Intercession on hotlines may need only sensitivity and an ability to calm a person in stress. But prevention?

14.5.3   Coronial Knowledge

New South Wales coroners told us that they learn on the job. Victoria's coroners have a collegial unit where they educate themselves and learn from each other. Law students don't have a curriculum unit on coronial law and practice. Nor do medical students, social workers, police, or hospital executives and staff. In order 'to speak of the dead to protect the living', one has to know a little something about the dead and their manner of dying. While the eminent Professor Joseph Zubin once said that it is nigh impossible to unravel the cause of a suicidal death, forensic anthropologists can reconstruct enough to give an outline of a temperament and a set of circumstances. Publishing such profiles, anonymously of course, is more likely to assist those in despair, and their families, than slogans?

14.5.4   The Role of Review

Herbert Simon (1916–2001) was a Nobel Economics Laureate and a giant in the field of administrative behaviour, the title of his 1947 masterpiece. He wrote eloquently on the nature and purpose of review, that is, the means by which the hierarchy learns whether decisions are being made correctly or incorrectly and whether work is being done well or badly at the lower levels. It is the fundamental source of information upon which the higher levels of an organisation can make decisions, learn and improve. First, it leads to a diagnosis of the quality of decisions being made by subordinates. Second, it leads to an influencing of subsequent decisions. Third, it assists in the correction of things that have gone wrong. Fourth, it is essential for the effective exercise of authority; it can only be applied if there is some means of ascertaining when authority has been respected and when it has been disobeyed (Simon 1950: 233–238).

Universities tend to engage external reviewers of a department or a discipline every three or five years. Department stores often do weekly reviews of how a product has fared. Some government agencies are reviewed only after an election. Whether it be audit in a financial sense or review in an effectiveness of goal-achievement sense, review by independent inspectors is preferable to an eventual judicial inquiry or royal commission.

Our concluding thoughts are that we need two reviews sooner than later: one is a review of the financing and effectiveness of prevention agencies; the other is an in-depth and critical look at social attitudes to suicide. We believe they need to change.

14.5.5 The Sports Factor

Oscar Wilde (1854–1900), the Irish poet, once wrote that 'rugby is a game for barbarians played by gentlemen. Football [soccer] is a game for gentlemen played by barbarians'. No matter the state of civilisation or the degree of civility involved, sport is one of our best forms of attraction and distraction. Not least is the excitement aroused in and by a crowd, the 'enemy' posed by the side opposing your team, the heavy expectation about the outcome, the voyeuristic combat, the vicarious imagination that it is you scoring the goal.

In 1981, the British zoologist Desmond Morris wrote *The Soccer Tribe*, relating the origins and rituals of the 'gentleman's' game. At its base, soccer derives from tribal affiliations, and if not from the primeval swamps then in Britain in about 1863, offering zealous support for places like Notts County, Sheffield Wednesday and Stoke City. Whatever it may be, the round ball game is the major universal sport, the one with an astonishing fan base. It is fandom, crowd fandom and fanaticism that makes for a protector against aloneness, alienation—and for a desire to see out the week, the year. It is the future tense of sport that negates the suicider's predicament of yesterday and today.

14.5.6 Critical Suicidology

Critical suicide studies have fundamental objections to the pathologising and medicalising of suicide. That approach flies in the face of history. But it also defies medical orthodoxies in that it persists with a 'treatment' that doesn't work for a 'disease' that it doesn't understand. Worse, it rejects other than its own insights and perspectives and does so in a manner that is certain, adamant, assertive, and with more than a touch of arrogance in its ignorance.

On a positive note, some psychiatrists and adjunct professions have now moved to a position that suicide can only be approached in a holistic way, that is, through multi-agency approaches. In Western Australia, Patricia Dudgeon and Tracey Westerman have shown how much can be done with empathetic Aboriginal cultural values and traditional psychology. They recognise context and the limitations of the biomedical model (see http://www.indigenouspsychology.com.au). The critical suicide movement constantly seeks a wider perspective, a holistic approach, lateral thinking: it offers a much broader vision of suicide than we have at present.

14.6   In Sum

14.6.1   The Suicide Enigma

Suicide is a compound of contradictions. It is a self-selected and self-inflicted premature death—'before one's time is up', an early surcease when long life is a prized social goal. Suicide is one's 'final freedom', an exercise of sovereignty over what may be the only asset the deceased may own. It ends the pain of one and causes pain to many. Once honoured, even celebrated, it is now pejorative, shaming, odious, softened by its portrayal as mental illness and thus 'excusable'.

Suicide is a social reality, but the response to it is a social construct. Are societal reactions inflated, over-emphasised, magnified, especially when compared to other forms of death? Is it a matter of control: there is little or nothing we can do to stop the metastasising cancer cell, to defeat the Ebola virus, in a victim who wants to live, but can we keep alive a person who doesn't want to be?

References

Barnard, C. (1949). *Organization and management: Selected papers*. Boston: Harvard University Press.
Battin, M. P. (2015). *The ethics of suicide: Historical sources*. Oxford: Oxford University Press.
Bering, J. (2018). *Suicidal: Why we kill ourselves*. Chicago: Chicago University Press.
Crosby, A. E., & Sacks, J. J. (2002). Exposure to suicide: Incidence and association with suicidal ideation and behavior, United States 1994. *Suicide and Life Therapy Behavior, 3,* 321–328.
Dervic, K., Oquendo, M., Grunebaum, M., & Mann, J. (2004). Religious affiliation and suicide attempts. *American Journal of Psychiatry, 161*(12), 2303–2308.
Durkheim, É. [1897] (2013). *Suicide: A study in sociology*. New York: The Free Press.
Eugenides, J. (1993). *The virgin suicides*. London: Farrar, Strauss and Giroux.
Hanna, J. (2017). Suicide under age 13: One every 5 days. CNN Health, 14 August.
Ireland, W. (1898). *The mental affections of children: Idiocy, imbecility and insanity*. London: J. and A. Churchill.
Marx, E. (1976). *The social context of violent behaviour: A social study of an Israeli immigrant town*. London: Routledge & Kegan Paul.

Morris, D. (1981). *The soccer tribe*. London: Jonathan Cape.

Peter, L., & Hull, R. (1969). *The Peter principle*. New York: William Morrow and Co.

Pritchard, C. (1995). *Suicide—The ultimate rejection?: A psycho-social study*. London: The Open University Press.

(RACGP) Royal Australian College of General Practitioners. (2018). *Health of the nation*. Melbourne.

Simon, H. (1950). *Adminstrative behavior: A study of decision-making processes in administrative organization*. New York: MacMillan Company.

Tollefsen, I. M., Hem, E., & Ekeberg, O. (2012). The reliability of suicide statistics: A systematic review. *BMC Psychiatry, 12*(9).

Appendix

There are three kinds of lies: lies, damed lies, and statistics.
—Benjamin Disraeli, or perhaps Mark Twain[1]

Suicide Rates for Forty-One Nations, 2017
Deaths per 100,000 of a population

1. Lithuania—26,700
2. Korea—25,800
3. Russia—19,300
4. Slovenia—18,100
5. Latvia—18,100
6. Japan—16,600
7. Hungary—16,200
8. Belgium—15,800
9. Estonia—14,100
10. United States—13,800
11. Poland—13,500
12. Finland—13,100
13. France—13,100
14. Australia—12,800
15. Switzerland—12,500
16. Austria—12,200
17. Iceland—12,100
18. New Zealand—11,800
19. Czech Republic—11,700
20. Sweden—11,200

---

[1]Disraeli was British prime minister and writer (1801–1884); Mark Twain was a famed American novelist and wit (1835–1910).

© Springer Nature Switzerland AG 2019
C. Tatz and S. Tatz, *The Sealed Box of Suicide*,
https://doi.org/10.1007/978-3-030-28159-5

21. Canada—11,100
22. Luxembourg—11,100
23. Norway—11,100
24. Chile—10,700
25. Germany—10,600
26. Ireland—10,600
27. Netherlands—10,500
28. Portugal—10,200
29. Slovak Republic—9,700
30. Denmark—9,400
31. United Kingdom—7,500
32. Spain—6,900
33. Brazil—6,000
34. Italy—5,700
35. Costa Rica—5,700
36. Mexico—5,500
37. Colombia—5,300
38. Israel—4,900
39. Greece—4,400
40. Turkey—2,100
41. South Africa—1,000

Source https://data.oecd.org/healthstat/suicide-rates.htm.

Index

A

Aboriginal autonomy, 90
Aboriginal deaths in custody, 62, 85
Aboriginal 'intervention', 90
Aboriginal suicide, 28, 64, 67, 85, 86, 90, 149, 156, 178, 194
Abstaining suicide, 63
Accidental suicide, 63
Acedia, 39
Active euthanasia, 128
Advance Directive/living will, 127
Advisory Centre for the Weary of Life (Vienna), 98
African slaves, 11
Aggressive suicide genre, 60
Alberti, Michael, 42
Alcohol/alcoholism and suicide, 32
Alcoholism, 105
Alienation, 11, 48, 61, 163–165, 186, 192, 195, 197
Alleviating/alleviation of suicide, 4, 163, 192
Allocation of responsibility functions, 173
Altruistic suicide, 36, 60, 61, 83
Alvarez, Al, 12, 13, 21, 24, 33, 34, 40, 67, 81
Amateurs, 146, 151, 152, 157, 171
Ambiguity concept, 126, 194, 195
American Indian and Alaska Mental Health Research Center, 92
American Indians, 79, 80, 86, 92, 102
American Medical Association, 130
American Psychiatric Association, 22, 23, 50, 158
Améry, Jean, 8, 37, 60, 62, 66, 67, 84
Anaesthetists, 48, 68, 158–160
Andrews, Kevin, 136

Anomic suicide, 60, 62, 68
Anorexia nervosa, 63
Anovak, Jack, 81
Antenatal and postnatal depression, 47
Anthropology, 3, 20, 28, 33, 92, 194
Anti-anxiety medications, 55
Antidepressants, 6, 25, 26, 43, 45–47, 53–55, 73–75, 81, 89, 99, 108, 109, 146, 155, 182
Anti-psychotic medications, 55
Anti-stigma campaigns, 28, 111
Anti-Suicide Bureau (UK), 97
Anti-Suicide League (Zurich), 98
Anxiety, 41, 43, 45, 47, 55, 101, 160, 165, 182, 183, 185, 186
Appealing suicide, 67
Aquinas, St Thomas, 10, 37
Armenian Apostolic Church, 83
Armenian genocide, 82, 83
Armenian women, 62, 66, 82, 83
Arson, 71
Art, 173
Art and suicide, 4
Asphyxiation, 71, 73
Aspirin, 45, 46, 56
Assimilation, 87, 88, 91, 157
Assistant coroners, 141
Assisted dying, 8, 20, 85, 125–127, 132–135, 181, 183, 188, 189
Assisted suicide, 7
Asylum-seekers, 62, 180, 190
Athletic participation and suicide, 169
At-risk factors, 28, 32, 93
Auschwitz, 8, 84
Australian Aborigines, 33, 80
Australian Medical Association (AuMA), 130, 159

Printed by Printforce, the Netherlands